UNBECOMING

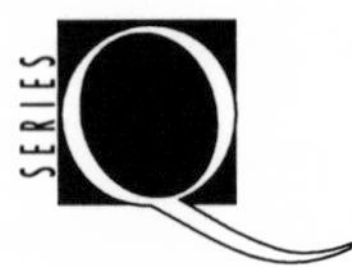

Edited by

Michèle Aina Barale,

Jonathan Goldberg,

Michael Moon, and

Eve Kosofsky Sedgwick

UNBECOMING *by Eric Michaels*

EDITED BY PAUL FOSS

NEW PREFACE BY MICHAEL MOON

INTRODUCTION BY SIMON WATNEY

DUKE UNIVERSITY PRESS *Durham 1997*

Printed in the United States of America on acid-free paper ∞
Typeset in Scala by Wilsted & Taylor Publishing Services
Library of Congress Cataloging-in-Publication Data
appear on the last printed page of this book.

In Memory of Terry Bell, Hugh Steers, and Dr. Richard Kemp

CONTENTS

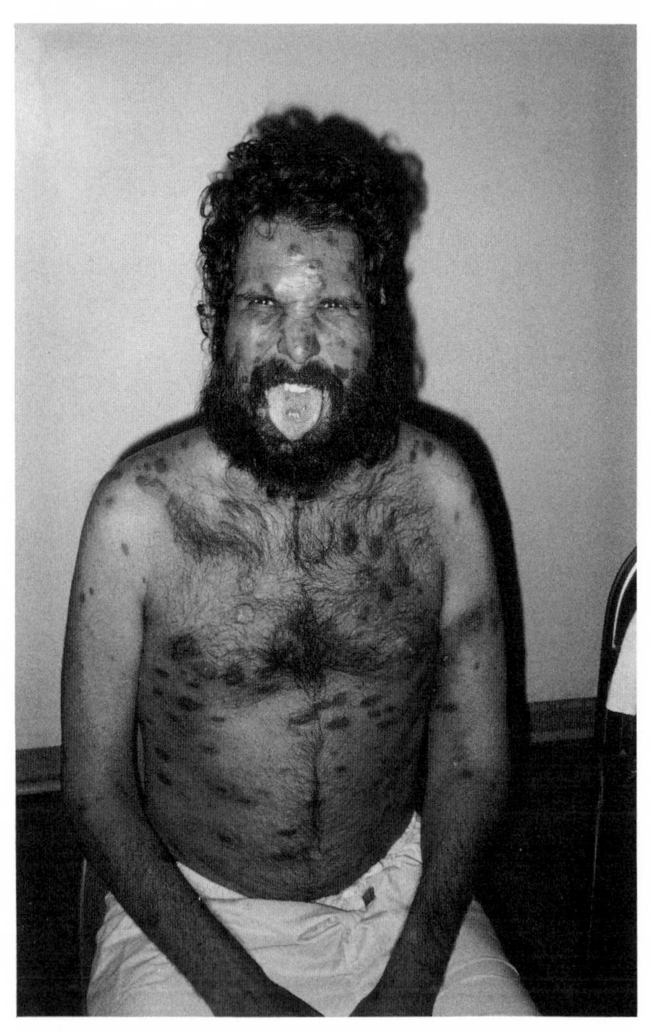

Eric Michaels, Brisbane, June 26, 1988.
Photo by Penny Taylor

PREFACE TO THE DUKE EDITION

Michael Moon

Almost all the major events and achievements of Eric Michaels's career are compressed into the middle years of a single decade, the 1980s, with a kind of brutality that AIDS has made painfully common. Nearly everything he published—several monographs and twenty-odd articles—appeared in the last four or five years of his life (i.e., 1984–88). Two volumes of Michaels's writing have appeared since his death: *Bad Aboriginal Art: Tradition, Media, and Technological Horizons,* which collects ten of his articles on the painting and television of the Warlpiri Aborigines of Western Central Australia, and the present volume, Michaels's "AIDS Diary," which he kept from 9 September 1987 to 10 August 1988 (he died on 24 August).

Michaels was a U.S. citizen who left the States in 1982, aged thirty-four, with a recent Ph.D. in anthropology from the University of Texas at Austin, to accept a job in Australia studying the uses of televisual technology by Aboriginal communities. Having rapidly established a reputation for himself as a formidable analyst of transcultural representations, he was teaching at Griffith University in Brisbane when, late in the summer of 1987, the symptoms of his illness began to present themselves. Here the diary begins. As a person living with AIDS, Michaels records his struggles with the immigration authority of the Australian government, with a health-care system ill-equipped to deal with AIDS, with academic bureaucracy, with successive landlords and neighbors, with the local gay community, with colleagues and a handful of friends in Brisbane and Sydney, with his family back in the States, and with drastic fluctuations in his own physical condition. The diary is full of Michaels's rage and frustration; it is also full of a wild kind of humor that can, under extreme circumstances, be the heart's only alternative to feeling—to paraphrase Swift's epitaph—lacerated by indignation. The furious letters Michaels wrote to the people and agencies that had treated him most shabbily during his final illness are charged with both an anger and a delight in his own wit under fire that are sharper than one can imagine almost any other feeling being, except the grief—his, ours—that sometimes seems to pool at the edge of the page, threatening to overwhelm Michaels's world and his affordance to his readers of a rich, if partial and temporary, relation to it.

Unbecoming provides valuable testimony about the emotional sources of a notable instance of what one might call "the will to theorize"—even, in Michaels's case, almost unto death. To his and our profit, he never stops thinking and theorizing about the determinants of his situation as an emphatically displaced person with AIDS, and rarely in a way that seems to abstract that situation, but rather in one that continually recurs to intractable but not unthinkable realities. Michaels launches a venomous tirade against the Australian cult of tidiness—a regional subvariant of what Eve Kosofsky Sedgwick has called "the hygienic imperative" in modern cultures—in his diary entry for 5–20 November, as he experienced it in the Infectious Diseases Ward of the Royal Brisbane Hospital. Despite the continual floor-buffing the beleaguered custodial staff is required to do, Michaels sees the inherent messiness and griminess of life and illness more than holding their own against the absurd, halfhearted, institutionalized wish to polish our troubles away.

In his foreword to this volume, Michaels's friend and sometimes publisher, Paul Foss, provides readers a few precious glimpses into the space that Mary Shelley memorably calls "the filthy workshop of creation," briefly but suggestively mentioning such non-academic pursuits of Michaels's as his work on *Suck* magazine in the days of "the rise and fall of Gay Liberation" and his "typically" (for the time) "nomadic screwball existence" in New York and New Mexico. When we speculate about how and why Michaels's published work on the deployment of electronic media among some Aboriginal communities—to many of us, a highly specialized and even esoteric-sounding topic—has come to be taught in courses in communications, cultural studies, film and video production, and postcolonial theory, throughout Australia and far beyond it, we should surely try to take into account his extra-academic experiences as a member of some of the most creative and volatile of the subcultures that proliferated in the late sixties and early seventies.

Even during the years he spent far from academia, Michaels remained a voracious, impassioned student and theorist of his life and culture. Early on in this diary he writes about having acquired "a gutful of psychologizing" as a "gifted child" and then a "troubled" adolescent from an affluent family who "had spent rather a lot of time in testing and therapy sessions" before he was twenty. "These sessions," he writes, "introduced me to a bewildering universe of praise and blame, obligation and independence which seemed quite impossible." "What was being reinforced," he goes on,

> was an extreme and alienating sense of my personal uniqueness, the vast gulfs which separated me from any other humankind. Thus, my encounter with culturalogical explanation was a revelation, a discovery embraced longingly. (17 September 1987)

The field of anthropology, "as taught in the U.S., circa 1966," the year he turned eighteen, provided the young Michaels with his first chance to think of himself not as uniquely and ineffably set apart, but as a "hypertypical" person, given the social and cultural forces he saw acting on and through himself and many of his generation. He used his postgraduate studies at the University of Texas to explore widely divergent aspects of the cultural politics of his place and time: he wrote a master's thesis on the dispersal of property among gay lovers, followed by a dissertation on the interpretation of television messages by local Christian-fundamentalist media-protest groups.

Michaels considered his being gay "the most dramatic example" in his own experience of what he saw as his hypertypicality as a person.

> I am convinced that had I been born only twenty years earlier (or maybe, twenty years later) I probably would not have been gay. Now, that's logically preposterous; 20 years' difference and I wouldn't have been "I." (Indeed, I have trouble with "I"-ness at

> every moment and writing is no cure for that at all.) . . . The homosexual world of the 1950s and early 1960s in a city such as Philadelphia [where Michaels grew up] remained constricted, marginal, inverted, covert. By contrast, in New York, 1971, "gay" was something impossibly chic, central to the cultural life of the city, a public rather than private form. . . . (17 September 1987)

This was written at the onset of an international wave of AIDS activism that radically transformed gay life in many places. Several years earlier, in 1982, Michaels had written an extraordinary, thousand-word statement/manifesto which is appended to the present text as its "endnote." In this text, composed at a historical moment when he felt that gay political activism had reached an apogee, Michaels laments the "deterioration" of "the movement" and the degradation of decades of gay subcultural life into a series of "niche" markets for "Nautilus, EST, and Coors Beer." For Michaels in 1982 the baseline truth about the decline of gay culture is that "we're not avant-garde anymore. We're not avant anything. We imitate everybody else now. They don't imitate us."

This issue of imitability and the power to compel imitation in others is at the core of Michaels's thinking, about matters as diverse as transcultural and transracial representation and the relative vitality or moribundity of gay cultural life. As Michaels observes in his diary entry for 9 February 1988, "Allen Ginsberg used to date the shift from Beat to Hippy as a shift from Black to Amerindian cultural imitation among white youth." Michaels goes on to argue contra Ginsberg that African-American culture never ceased to serve as the primary object of imitation for young white Americans who aspired to be "cool" in the late sixties and afterward.

While puzzling over the meanings of the absence of such a model among his white Australian contemporaries, Michaels's thinking manifests a momentary blindspot about the histories of their and his relations to Aboriginal peoples. This acute critic of the politics of transcultural exchange nowhere, neither in his professional anti-ethnographic writing nor in his diary, makes an explicit inventory of his obvious indebtedness to the Warlpiri Aborigines, although when he does write about them in his diary, it is with the unmistakable tone of affectionate and respectful regard with which one speaks of only one's best and truest teachers. It is from these associates, for example, that Michaels mentions having learned that a person has strong and unarguable claims on the place where he or she is going to die. Sitting in the bath on 17 March 1988, Michaels imagines being criticized on the radio for attempting (successfully) to "pass" as a lifelong Australian in the celebrated article on Sydney's Gay Mardi Gras he had just written. He imagines replying:

> As is true of so many here, I was not born in Australia; one has little choice in these matters. But it appears I will die here. My first teachers of Australianism, the old Warlpiri men of Yuendumu, believe that fact gives me certain rights here, which I am entitled to invoke.

At such moments, Michaels's writing anticipates some of the very fertile work in cultural studies done in the years since his death on the phenomenon of cross-identification, across race and ethnicity, nationality, class, gender, and sexuality. The possibility of complex and many-sided, multidirectional and asymmetrical processes of identification and "imitation" has been much enriched by the theories and practices of critical race studies, gender and queer studies, and the focus of postcolonial studies on subaltern positions and non- and antinational cultural and political formations. "Autoethnography" is one of the terms that has been circulated and debated in recent years on the part of some theorists championing certain forms of communal knowledge that are, to invoke Michaels's terms for his own intellectual awakening in the mid-sixties, both "culturalogical" and "anti-psychologistic." Of the strong critiques on received notions of the "ethnographic" and its intellectual and cultural privileges that have been made over the past twenty-five years, Michaels's attacks on prevailing assumptions about the uses and abuses of ethnographic film and video have proven to be some of the most devastating. In his AIDS diary, Michaels pays the cost (literally, since he directed that his small estate be used to defray the costs of the first publication of his diary) of his passionate belief that the self was precious principally because it provided a point of epistemological entry into the realm of "culturalogical" hypertypicality, where a larger weather prevailed than that of the ego and its very limited range of obsessions.

Michaels's writing is also valuable for the ways in which it reveals how certain ideas and desires currently associated with queer theory have circulated in gay and lesbian discourse in earlier forms. The complex connections between lesbian and gay identities and performativity, the critique of "essentialist" conceptions of gender and sexuality—these and other related notions inform Michaels's work at many points, as they have informed much fine work in the years since his death. In his article on Gay Mardi Gras (reprinted in the present volume under the entry for 17 March 1988), for example, Michaels delights in the thorough confusion of the imaginary "line" between gay and straight participants in the outrageous rites of carnivale as he sees them being reinvented in the streets of Sydney. Against those who would argue that gays and lesbians represent a new "ethnic community" in the Australian melting-pot, he argues that a more serviceable analogy might be made "to the medieval guilds, collectivities of craft, residence, and ideology which staged the original Carnivales."

The collective autoethnographies Michaels exemplarily improvises—for gays and lesbians, for persons with AIDS—tend to range far, both historically (medieval guilds) and geographically (the old Warlpiri men of Yuendumu). Michaels, already a severe critic of some of the institutions of therapy and self-development in his teens, was exceptional among our generation of precocious readers of the bildungsroman—*The Red and the Black, Père Goriot, A Sentimental Education, Portrait of a Lady, Daniel Deronda, The Way of All Flesh, Portrait of the Artist, The Magic Mountain, The Voyage Out, Remembrance of Things Past, The Longest Journey*—in bringing much in the way of resistance to its seductive teleologies. Studying to become "somebody," cultivating what we considered to be a rich subjectivity, amassing intellectual and cultural capital in its many forms, was for a long time the driving force in the lives of many of the more privileged of those of us born within a decade or so on either side of Michaels's birth in 1948. When Paul Foss visits Michaels in the hospital in November 1987 and reads some of the early drafts of his diary, his response (a "hypertypical" one for someone of our age and social class) is to devise a reading project for Michaels on the spot, with an extensive improvised bibliography. If Michaels is going to keep an "AIDS diary," he must read Defoe (presumably *A Journal of the Plague Year*) and Gide's and Joe Orton's diaries. An instant trip to the hospital bookstore yields only *The Diary of Anne Frank*. "Guided reading till you drop" was a comic watchword among overtutored undergraduates in elite American colleges in the sixties; it lives on as a kind of calcified reflex for many of us.

What Michaels did not live to see, although he does in his diary foresee the conditions that will enable it, is the making of ample market niches in the decade since his death for a whole range of "AIDS cultural commodities": the AIDS play, the AIDS novel, poem, diary, movie, magazine, and so on. As works in these mostly melancholy subgenres, some superbly powerful, many "no better than they should be," continue to proliferate, at least for a while longer, Michaels's AIDS writing will remain useful and necessary for the intensely high level of clear-eyed rage it brings to bear on the role that one typical national health system plays in increasing the anguish of one avowedly "hypertypical" person struggling to deal with a debilitating illness. It may serve some members of our generation and the subsequent one well in this ongoing and difficult phase of our thorough, if unheralded, unexpected, and mostly unwanted, education in dispossession, in "unbecoming."

Note

I wish to thank Julie Graham of the University of Massachusetts at Amherst and Kathy Gibson of Monash University, Melbourne, for recommending *Unbecoming: An AIDS Diary* to me, and Ross Chambers of the University of Michigan for recommending it to Eve Kosofsky Sedgwick. Thanks also to Paul Foss for the care he has lavished on the text of this new edition of *Unbecoming*. Conversations with Eve, Jonathan Goldberg, Lauren Berlant, and Michael Warner have been enormously helpful to me in thinking about the significance of Eric Michaels's writing in the larger context of the history of the transmission of queer culture through the past several decades.

FOREWORD

Paul Foss

Eric Michaels, American-born analyst of Central Australian Aboriginal TV, and lecturer in media studies at Griffith University, died from AIDS in a Brisbane hospital on the morning of 24 August 1988. He was just forty. He left behind these occasional journals that were destined to recount only the last year of his life, and for which he offered, should they be published, the title *Unbecoming.*

It has taken some years to get the diary into print,[1] involving many people from the critical and artistic circles of Sydney, Canberra, and Brisbane. Without the assistance of Penny Taylor, John von Sturmer, Stuart Cunningham, and Liz Fell—to single out just the principal readers and supporters of the diary (though here I should also mention Terry Bell, Ross Harley, and Paul Paech)—this publication would not have appeared. My own role has simply been to coordinate all this shared labor on behalf of someone we all deeply admired, both as a friend and through respect for his work.

Eric Michaels was trained as an anthropologist before coming to Australia in late 1982. A postgraduate at the University of Texas, he did his masters on the dispersal of property among gay lovers, followed by a doctorate on the social organization of the interpretation of TV messages in a small Texas city, which was based on fieldwork with Protestant fundamentalist media protest groups. Yet these academic pursuits were not unconnected to the life he'd led during the late 1960s and early 1970s. A nice, Jewish, white boy born and bred in the bluestocking belt of America's eastern seaboard, the young Eric had gone AWOL—as anyone with good looks and style did in those heady, fuck-anything days. He witnessed the rise and fall of Gay Liberation in New York; was involved with *Suck* magazine; joined an art gallery co-op in Philadelphia; ran a macrobiotic store; resided in New Mexican communes for a time; and, all told, led a typically nomadic screwball existence before taking up his studies at Austin, Texas.

After finishing his doctorate, Eric accepted a fellowship from the Australian Institute of Aboriginal Studies in Canberra to research the impact of television on remote Aboriginal communities—eventually published as *The Aboriginal Invention of Television, 1982–86* (Canberra: AIAS, 1986). He remained in the Central/Western Desert region where he involved himself in claims by various Aboriginal media associations for increased local autonomy in video production and circulation (cf. "Aboriginal Content: Who's Got It—Who Needs It?" [*Art & Text* 23–24, 1987], and *For a Cultural Future: Francis Jupurrurla Makes TV at Yuendumu* [Melbourne: Art & Criticism Monograph Series, vol. 3, 1988]). At the same time, Eric became interested in the new acrylic "dot paintings" carried out at Yuendumu and Papunya, occasioning the essays "Western Desert Sandpainting and Postmodernism" (in Warlukurlangu Artists, *Kuruwarri: Yuendumu Doors* [Canberra: AIAS, 1987]) and "Bad Aboriginal Art" (*Art & Text* 28, 1988). With these writings, exemplary in their refusal to romanticize indigenous cultures, Eric gained a wide following in Australia for his non-ethnographic approach to Aboriginal video and art.[2]

In early 1987 Eric accepted a teaching position at Griffith University in Brisbane, even though it was dependent upon the renewal of his resident status. This was eventually blocked by the Queensland Department of Immigration once it realized he had AIDS, despite interventions on his behalf by colleagues, doctors, and other government officials. Hounded by Immigration to the very end, he found himself quarantined in hospital under direct threat of expulsion from the country.

The diary traces this looming imbroglio. Here is the account of someone interrogating his failure to find a place to which he could devote himself, the city that had ensnared him, and the state he felt had ignored his labors. No one is spared in these pages. Close friends and relatives, Brisbane drivers, bureaucrats, academics, hospital staff, Australian TV programming, even the neighbors who hogged the communal clothesline—all are treated to Eric's unique, often hilarious brand of acrimony.

Yet it is impossible to situate, let alone express, the narrative's true state of mind. Even accepting Eric's deep sense of loss and betrayal, how we might end up regarding the diary requires, at the very least, far more than pathos or community outrage. For behind all the venom and impish reverie, there's a crucial issue here: not just dying, at some time, in some place, but dying a death for which no ceremony or lament has prepared us, where no ground awaits, no "spirit" to call, no etiquette, taboo, or, dare one say it, *veneration*—nothing but that blank indifference shown a glob of spittle or dung heap, something unutterably alien and formless. What else is left, as Gary Indiana writes in *Horse Crazy* (1989), but to "become hypnotized by the disappearance of yourself"?

In the end, I believe Eric is challenging us not only to communicate his lot to others, but also to question our social compact, our rituals of exchange, that "full" body of sociality in which he found himself implanted like a germ—deforming, in a fashion, the solidity and cohesiveness of our culture's belief systems, just as the virus was dissolving his integrity of form. This was not through spite, but because he genuinely believed in the sovereignty of diverse peoples and their cultural practices, in those specific rites of passage by which everyone, whatever creed, color, or taste, defines and negotiates the sum total of existence. For how each of us chooses to die, or live, ultimately influences the fate of us all.

Gay artist David Wojnarowicz describes it best in "Postcards from America" (1989), and in a manner which seems to me to come closest to the cry of exasperation uttered by Eric in those horrifying last days in Brisbane: "WHEN I WAS TOLD THAT I'D CONTRACTED THIS VIRUS IT DIDN'T TAKE ME LONG TO REALIZE THAT I'D CONTRACTED A DISEASED SOCIETY AS WELL."

Notes

1 This preface is a modified version of the one published in the first edition of *Unbecoming* (Sydney: EMPress, 1990). For the new edition, the diary has been corrected and expanded to include "Carnivale in Oxford St." A bibliography of the

works of Eric Michaels may be found in his posthumous anthology, *Bad Aboriginal Art: Tradition, Media, and Technological Horizons* (Minneapolis: University of Minnesota Press, 1994).

2 For these essays as well as critical evaluations of Michaels's work, see *Bad Aboriginal Art.* Further discussion may be found in the special issue, "Communication & Tradition: Essays after Eric Michaels," *Continuum* 3:2 (Perth, 1990).

INTRODUCTION

Simon Watney

Wars are no longer waged in the name of a sovereign who must be defended; they are waged on behalf of the existence of everyone; entire populations are mobilized for the purpose of wholesale slaughter in the name of life necessity: massacres have become vital.—Michel Foucault[1]

I am so frightened that the war against AIDS has already been lost.
—Larry Kramer[2]

There is now a considerable and growing testimonial literature of AIDS, mainly written from the subject-positions of people living with the self-conscious effects—both social and clinical—of having been infected by the Human Immunodeficiency Virus (HIV). In fiction, poetry, and autobiography, people living with AIDS have attempted to flesh out their experiences and feelings for an audience that is generally presumed to be uninfected. Running right across this literature is the metaphor of war. "The war against AIDS" has been conceived in many ways, ranging from the need for a new Manhattan Project in the field of biomedical research, to wars on behalf of adequate safer-sex education, welfare rights, and so on. It is however still only rarely perceived that HIV and AIDS were long hence mobilized to the purposes of another struggle, moreover a struggle that has been taking place with growing ferocity throughout the modern period. This war concerns the power of the state to define "the public good," frequently in terms of "public health." From this perspective the systematic denials of adequate health education and care and the directions of international research make perfect, coherent sense. For the "war against AIDS" has never principally targeted HIV, or its multiple, tragic consequences in the lives of individuals or communities. On the contrary, from the perspective of the state, it has been precisely and skillfully targeted against those of whom an AIDS diagnosis is held to reveal a far more deadly threat that reaches to the very heart of the epistemology of modernity, and the compliant identities it lovingly nurtures within the strict categories of gender, race, and sexuality.[3]

I never met Eric Michaels but was aware like many others of his distinguished work as an anthropologist and critic. As his remarkable AIDS diary reveals, he was well aware of the ironic relation between his life's work and the public meanings generated around the syndrome that eventually killed him. In one of his most justly celebrated papers, he described how

> [t]he way that Warlpiri people talk about paintings and designs revolves around . . . questions of authority. Who owns the design? Who may see it? Who is authorized to paint (reproduce) it?[4]

Such questions concerning the rights (and representations) of people living with HIV and AIDS have proved fundamental to the emergent cultural politics of the epidemic—a politics that recognizes the active role played by processes of representation at all levels in the management of all aspects of social policy, from health promotion to the directions of biomedical research, and service provision. Yet the "authenticity" of an HIV or AIDS diagnosis guarantees nothing by way of the supposed truth status of the testimonial literature of AIDS. We have seen and heard enough people with AIDS castigating themselves on television or in the press for the imaginary crimes of "promiscuity," or "sex addiction," or whatever, to be skeptical of the familiar sickroom diary format. Besides, who would choose to be a speaking virus? Certainly not Eric Michaels.

Hence he invites us to identify with his physical perception of his bed in the infectious diseases ward of Royal Brisbane Hospital as a place where

> multiple lines of discourse converge, like ley lines converge at Stonehenge. A person lying in my bed merely looking round the room and out the window can see great distances, to parliamentary debates on condoms and morals, to histories of Australian asylums, etiquettes, hierarchies, and colonialisms. But what most has me flat on my back here is a discourse of "Tidiness."

Michaels rages at the pettiness of the colonized variants of British hyperdomesticity, thus revealing much of his American identity. Indeed, perhaps only an American leftist of his generation could fail to recognize the absurdity (and callousness) of dismissing Joe Orton as a "class traitor." Yet his wonderfully splenetic revenge letters also suggest the extent to which he had taken on the familiar passive-aggressive characteristics of Australian-mediated Englishness. It is, after all, deeply refreshing to discover someone who so dearly loathed his mother. Yet he is never unself-knowing. For example, he points out acutely that 1968 *did* lead to a revolution, in relation to the subsequent politics of race and gender. He also openly acknowledges the extent to which he deliberately provoked crises in other people, though one would forgive much in a man whose implacable hatred of Paul Simon is dated so specifically to "I Am A Rock" in 1966.

Eric Michaels was evidently a gritty, stubborn, difficult man. How else could he recognize that

> [i]t is the profound moral imperatives and ethical calculations which ultimately do drive great gay queens throughout this century (and the last, as far as it can be determined).

It was this intellectual strength which informs his relentless depiction of his own work within a hospital system that evidently wished him dead. It is constantly painful, and salutary, to witness him trying to think creatively through all the protracted stages in which the bureaucracy of his adopted and much loved/hated country did its damnedest to kick him out—right to the bitter end. For example, we are obliged to speculate about the relations between his charge that anthropologists may end up inventing the very people they purport to describe, and his parallel awareness as a gay man that gay politics aims deliberately and most specifically to create its own tribal identities and institutions. In such speculations his project will continue.

This edition of his AIDS diary ends with a remarkable, undated text on gay politics, which was probably written in 1982. It contains many of the man's enduring strengths and contradictions. For he was unusual not least in his keen ability to see himself and his generation of sixties gay activists—as they still are frequently regarded by subsequent generations. He notes that

> we conjure up an image in the minds of our younger friends of wild-eyed radical transvestites and hairy hippy faggots battling the forces of authority.

I do not happen to share his belief that a supposedly pure, leftist "gay political sensibility" was subsequently sold out by craven commercial and conservative interests. Nor do I find that the many young lesbians and gay men whom I frequently meet from all around the world are uniformly bent on becoming "accepted" as greedy yuppies. On the contrary, I agree with Michaels elsewhere in this same text, where he argues that older gay men

> need to take some responsibility for our own history, for conveying it to our young. It is not nostalgia. If one is going to go to all the trouble to be gay, one ought to do a more interesting and useful job of it. Models exist in our very recent past. They should be recalled.

I have little doubt that this was in large part the underlying motive behind his AIDS diary. If the young are indeed dismissive of what they associate with Gay Liberation, then this is only because they have had so little opportunity to understand their own immediate prehistory. This is one of the many reasons why the publication of Eric Michaels's diary matters, because it gives such immediate access to the cost of knowledge for his generation. And just as I agree that older gay men have a moral responsibility to the young, so it follows that they in time will recognize and assume their responsibility for us, or at least for those of us from the heyday of Gay Lib who happen to survive these terrible times. Nor is this a lesson which only gay men can learn, or should learn. For the war that this book exposes so eloquently and forcefully seems set to be *indefinite.*

Notes

1 Michel Foucault, *The History of Sexuality: An Introduction* (Harmondsworth: Penguin, 1981), 137.
2 Larry Kramer, "A 'Manhattan Project' for AIDS," *The New York Times* (16 July 1990).
3 See Simon Watney, "The Spectacle of AIDS," in *AIDS: Cultural Analysis, Cultural Activism*, ed. Douglas Crimp (Cambridge, Mass.: MIT Press, 1988).
4 Eric Michaels, "Bad Aboriginal Art," *Art & Text* 28 (March–May 1988), 71.

UNBECOMING

September 9, 1987

I watched these spots on my legs announce themselves over a period of weeks, taking them as some sort of morphemes, arising out of the strange uncertainties of the past few years to declare, finally, a scenario. As if these quite harmless-looking cancers might, when strung together, form sentences which would give a narrative trajectory, a plot outline, at last to a disease and a scenario that had been all too vague. Rather like when I was busted for speed and works with Horace and David, and thrown in that awful prison in Poughkeepsie, New York, in 1968. A moment's relief: it's come to this. The narrative, clear and insistent. Automatic pilot. But, of course, this relief proves always a false and premature dispensation. Perhaps the oddest thing about AIDS is that it takes so very long; one is required to live through all its stages, at each point confronted with insane, probably pathological choices. This week, it's who to tell, and how.

I rather like the choice to tell my computer, to engage in the curious restrictive circuit which makes electronic inscription seem such a narcissistic jerk-off. I don't much want to publicize my disease any further—but, of course, I will have to. So today, I told Stuart. I had thought the best thing would be to invite Stuart and Lee over for Sunday brunch so that we could have a group discussion; it seems rather a lot of responsibility to unload on a single friend what must yet remain secret. I thought this collective approach very smart indeed, only I ended up telling Stuart rather than merely extending the invitation for brunch. Now, I'm sitting at home typing instead of going over to his house for the big party he announced weeks ago, which I hope I didn't ruin, but to which I think it's probably better not going under the circumstances. What circumstances? Well, I'm not sure.

All this is a prelude to admitting the real difficulty, which is keeping such a journal, undertaking any diary at all. For whom do I write? And, worse yet, from what position? I could hedge and claim that I write for myself, in the hope that I can preserve for myself some clarity in a process which is likely to become very clouded very soon. And for myself, in the sense of a nearly biological drive to self-inscription which we recognize (but do not always forgive) at such moments. Do I imagine such a text will be read, or even published? Necessarily, a missive (missile) from the grave (which of course solves, or at least hijacks, the question of positioning). And what would be the rules governing the inscriptive practice here? Do I have to impose an orderly chronology? May I revise or not? Must I write every day, lest the precious residue of my thoughts be lost? . . . Or, how ever could one inflict such obligations on friends or readers, without requiring them to regard one as indulgent, foolish, perhaps bribing interest by inducement to trace in the prose deteriorations of judgment or style as a consequence of the deteriorating corpus? To elicit a truly grotty sympathy? I shall return to these morbid reflexivities repeatedly, I expect, through the course of . . . events? the disease? the plot? But not right now; right now these considerations exhaust me.

My point in taking hand to pen today, rather than next week or last, is mostly reportorial, to note simply that I have just today returned from two nights spent in the infectious diseases ward—curiously and deceptively named "Wattlebrae"—at the Royal Brisbane Hospital, which now houses AIDS patients. When I went in for tests on Wednesday evening, I should have realized, but didn't, that they would put me in such a place. Mama, you wouldn't believe how people treat you there! It's not the rubber gloves or face masks, or bizarre plastic wrapping on everything. It's the way people address you, by gesture, by eye, by mouth. And yet, done with the tests, I walk out on the street, go to work, and assume a comparatively normal interactive stance and distance. What begins here is a process of labeling, a struggle with institutional forms, a possible Foucauldian horror show, which must be resisted, counteracted somehow. I imagine that diary-keeping might serve to keep another set of definitions going against the quite barbaric ones that were inflicted in these last few days, through the rubber gloves, face masks, goggles, and an inventory of tropes assumed lately by medical practice to deal not so much with disease (which, after all, is imaginable in some sense as well), but more evidently, no less, with sin and retribution.

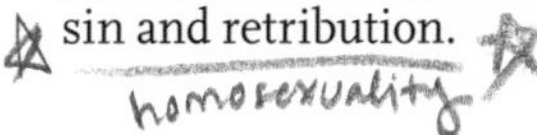

September 13, 1987

Richard, my doctor, has taken on the challenge to get me through to my 40th birthday. February: not a very long time.

What am I going to do with the books? The Aboriginal art? The photographs? For somebody intentionally bereft of the material, there does seem a lot to deal with. And worse, each of my possessions proves complex and complicated in terms that arise only now when faced with the prospect of dispersal. The logistics of all that seem impossible. Well, I'll deal with that tomorrow. The more immediate problem seems to be managing the sequence of disclosures.

Told Lee yesterday. . . . And he'd actually produced a lot of necessary information by tonight, and called me back. Went with Stuart and Jo to a public TV meeting and met all these people who want me to do one thing or another for them in the next few months, even years. I find it very odd to be discussing my keynote speech to the September 1988 Australian Teachers of Media Conference with the organizer. Called Paul F., who himself just got out of hospital (flu only, but something is suspicious, maybe just advanced hypochondria). I'm really quite taken with the opportunities to stage-manage all this: setting up my editor, my publisher, my archivist, etc. Which then seems to require that I stay up late making these precious diary entries. Stuff it; I'm going to sleep. I'm actually scheduled for five lectures this coming week. Altogether excessive in the best of circumstances.

September 17, 1987

I can't believe everybody doesn't have AIDS. I don't refer to any abstract calculations. In fact, I watch people very closely, especially their skin, for signs. I suspect celebrities on television most. Lots of them, we've always assumed, are gay. Does this explain Michael Jackson or Elton

John's bizarre behavior recently? But more, I watch moles on Cameron Daddo's face and consider Molly Meldrum's hair loss and pallor. It soon becomes clear that many people have moles, pimples, blemishes, discolorations: but these are not cancers, nor symptoms of AIDS. Why not? At first, I develop an obsessive erotic fantasy about flawless skin (this, in fact, dates from the psoriasis of last March). My pornographic magazine companions were subject to the closest inspections. Soon this reversed, so that I now limit my interest only to people with rough, flawed skin, finding porcelain blondes somewhat nauseating.

What is behind all this seems to be an anthropological calculation. In my youth, I had rather a gutful of psychologizing. Perhaps because it was the 1950s and America was inventing "gifted children" who could be bred to compete with the Russians and recover from the shame of Sputnik. Or perhaps it was because I exhibited certain characteristic sensibilities thought to make me vulnerable to deviancy. In any case, I had spent rather a lot of time in testing and therapy sessions by the time I was a college sophomore. These sessions introduced me to a bewildering universe of praise and blame, obligation and independence which seemed quite impossible to me. What was being reinforced was an extreme and alienating sense of my personal uniqueness, the vast gulfs that separated me from any other humankind. Thus, my encounter with culturalogical explanation was a revelation, a discovery embraced longingly. For anthropology (even more than sociology as taught in the U.S., circa 1966) seemed to argue against psychologism: the individual is a social/cultural collaborative construct, not an atomistic product of individual will. This produced in me a sense of enormous relief. For I always found suspicious my friends' belief in personal gods, beings who listened and responded to the prayers of each and every Protestant child. It made much more sense to me to see my "self" as socially constructed and culturally defined. The most dramatic example of this regards my sense of my homosexuality.

I am convinced that had I been born only 20 years earlier (or maybe, 20 years later), I probably would not have been gay. Now, that's logically preposterous; 20 years' difference and I wouldn't have been "I." (Indeed, I have trouble with "I"-ness at every moment and writing is no cure for that at all.) But the trope is convenient to illustrate my feeling that homosexual expression arises at particular moments in connection with other, dominant sexual and gender forms that are historically consequential, if not causal. As a youth, aware that I was capable of homosexual expression (or, more precisely, discovering that it evoked no guilt or other constraining mechanisms), I made some brief, protected incursions into the homosexual world but rejected what I found there: deviance. Whatever I might be, it was not what these people seemed; I could not be that isolated, that different. What I was seeking in my teen years was membership, a collective identity, my boy scout troop. The homosexual world of the 1950s and early 1960s in a city such as Philadelphia remained constricted, marginal, inverted, covert. By contrast, in New York, 1971, "gay" was something impossibly chic, central to the cultural life of the city, a public rather than private form, beginning to assume that enormous sense of importance that Western society would accord gayness in the 1970s while straights bungled their sexual politics and aesthetics. When I finally "came out," it was at New York parties reported in the next morning's papers, amongst famous, talented people.

What lurks behind all this is an unreconstructed 1960s sense of "where's it at" (happening now, baby!). I lived my life on those covers of *Life* magazine which identified and named trendy locales, the "in places," those ephemeral sites created by the contradictory explosions and implosions of the birth and death of the global village. I came close to a complete itinerary, so that my biography, if it were undertaken, might sound ridiculously like an epic fan magazine, or maybe Terry Southern's parody of Candide. In the process of these journeys, one sort of biographical self became somehow submerged, while another may have emerged in the residue of the first's assumption of the pretensions of Everyman. This is why I have AIDS, because it is now on the cover of *Life*, circa 1987. And this is why I can't believe that everyone doesn't have it, because of the sense in which I believe myself hypertypical. And if any of this is so, then it explains why the world I look out on now seems so dreary and painful, so devoid of joy, so mean and petty, not such a bad place to leave. The implications of an end to liberated sex and the death of gayness has truly miserable cultural/demographic/historical implications, even more than just a world of mean-minded hypocrites and wowsers shaking their fingers and saying, "I told you so." The reason I'm not terribly interested in living in such a world/future is not that it isn't any fun. I haven't had, nor sought, any fun since 1975. It's the oppressions, the cathedrals of inequality and greed that are to be built out of that rhetoric of the failure of liberation that I have no great wish to see.

September 20, 1987

Calvin sends me clippings from the San Francisco press describing the benefits of macrobiotics for PWAS and antibody-positives (I don't know whether San Francisco politically correct jargon identifies these as the same thing or not; Gary Cooper once sent me a letter suggesting I might be a "worried well" . . . the rhetoric may kill us before the virus!). Roger sends me similar clippings from Honolulu. Calvin says he is now macrobiotic. Paul calls me from Sydney to tell me to eat vegetables and quit smoking. Well, I did quit smoking, which I am assured St. Peter will note in my favor. But what is it with all these people? Are they antibody positive and not willing to tell me or anyone? Or are they unwilling to be tested and performing "as if" (an option I agree to politically but find personally/psychologically out of the question). Or, perhaps they are simply terribly concerned about me, and about other friends who may be in similar shape, involved in creating, at this late date, a kind of community or support network (get thee behind me, jargon!) in which who is sick and who isn't is precisely not the point (the position I hoped would emerge rather than the more general "every man for himself").

But circumstances now compel me to state, "Why I am not a macrobiotic"—which seems somewhat less grand than being Bertrand Russell and explaining why I am not a Christian, but we don't choose our times. I was once a macrobiotic. . . . (Inasmuch as several weeks later I found it necessary to severely restrict my diet along essentially macrobiotic lines, it seems silly to try and reconstruct this argument in reviewing/editing here.)

November 5–20, 1987

To celebrate the fifth anniversary of my arrival in Australia, I accepted an invitation to give a paper at Sydney University in the Anthropology Department on October 29, to be followed by a party thrown on the 31st. I offered the title "Bad Aboriginal Art" and then had to write something. It was hard work, especially because it had to be finished the same weekend I moved out of my impossible Kangaroo Point punk apartment into my New Farm "boojie" flat. I called the doc and checked to see if I could take some antibiotics with me to Sydney if I needed propping up. In fact, I felt lung congestion coming on and started the treatment even before I left. There was also a public TV conference, video editing for the Powerhouse Museum exhibit, text editing the Yuendumu monograph with Paul. . . . I staggered off the return plane to Brisbane on November 3, fell into bed, and checked into hospital the next day. I'd exhausted my body's tolerance to the antibiotic. In short, I'd wrecked myself. I'd wiped out my white blood cells (among others) and had no energy, no defense against anything, and was teetering on the edge. I was surrounded by people convinced I would die. It would be nearly a month before I got off my back, out of the hospital, and into my new flat. I insert these facts while editing. Obviously, I wasn't doing much writing at the time. And although I did bring the laptop into the hospital in a couple of weeks, these following entries are mostly undated. I was particularly concerned with the idea of writing a will. . . .

* * *

As with most other Aboriginal Australian peoples, the Warlpiri community I lived with at Yuendumu maintains elaborate, protracted mourning ceremonies. As dramatic as these are, they involve a contradiction in that, upon death, an individual's property, image, even name, must be obliterated. The camp is burned, people move away. Songs and designs belonging to the deceased exit the collective repertoire, sometimes for generations. Today, photographs, audio- and videotapes—all the modern forms of automatic inscription—must be obliterated or sealed away; it is more than a terrible insult to invoke the dead with recordings, it means trouble. Also, the name of the individuals, or more precisely, names associated with the deceased (Warlpiri naming practices and their epistemology resist any easy summary), go out of usage for roughly a generation. So do words deemed to sound like the name. These are forbidden to the common lexicon, and proscribed in discourse. The contradiction of course is that this all assures that a great deal of attention is actually directed toward the absence of this individual who we go to so much effort not to name. It is an elegant contradiction, however, very useful within its cultural context. Not only did I feel required to take these prohibitions into account with respect to my writing and publishing, as well as the very interesting implications of literacy here, I discovered that the idea became very sensible to me. For some time I refused to look at pictures of Rick, or of my mother, after they died, except surreptitiously. And of course, this poses a particular problem for my own work, and my relationship to the community which is the subject of so much of my writing. This, along with the disclosures, is one of those things I will have to muddle out, to produce in fact an analytic assessment of. My will, it seems, will be a position paper.

As far as I can tell, I have only intellectual property to dispense. Even here, the distinctive notions of property and the consequently contrasting practices of ownership on the one hand, and what might be called guardianship on the other, problematize utterly what's mine (to dispense) and what isn't. As for the matter of postmortem naming, for example, posthumous publication of my work, I see no problem. I am not, nor have I ever wanted or imagined myself to be, a Warlpiri Aboriginal. I come from a culture which honors the dead by invoking their names (i.e., trees in Israel, Washington's Vietnam War Memorial, or any local town square for that matter). I've no conviction that there persists after death any personal "me" in the least concerned about these things; indeed, my whole thinking resists utterly any such vulgar, ethnocentric, essentialist notions of personhood. Instead, I tell myself I'm looking forward to the rest. But I do imagine (and think the ethnography of many societies indicates) that there is created in a lifetime a sort of social body, perhaps something like what Gurdjieff meant by the soul—a persona which would exist outside the self, indeed become quite independent of it (what is Madonna really like?)—and that this obviously remains, as community property, for some time. I suppose, for whatever reasons, it is this being that I am investing so heavily in right now, perhaps in an attempt to honor/repay/justify friendships and family who are likely to mull over my life and death a good deal. I'd like to provide some interesting things to mull over, and not entirely morbid ones. But this requires my continued naming after death, and offends the Warlpiri custom. The issue may cause some pain at Yuendumu (not meaning to be presumptuous), but I expect some people will indeed feel "too sorry" to speak of me. I wonder whether Jupurrurla—on hearing of my death—will burn my Texas cowboy boots which I will send him next week, or whether, as I hope, he will find and invoke some dispensation, some loophole in the

"Law" to permit him to wear them for a while. For years, he eyed them with such obsessive fervor! It's these little researchable questions I'm a bit disappointed not to be able to test out any further.

But as for questions of property ownership or custodianship—I find I can't distance myself from them so easily, or invoke cross-cultural exemption. On reviewing my "property" today with the lawyer arranging my will, I had to admit I had almost none, or rather nothing of what most people would consider of value, economic or otherwise. There's a beat-up (but working) old car, currently out of registration that would be very hard to unload but might bring $1,500. That is the most valuable single thing I unequivocally "own." My library could be converted into a few thousand dollars cash by clever placement in specialist second-hand bookshops; but who wants to bother? Likewise, my Aboriginal art and artifacts (or what's left after the removalists robbed me of the best canvases) could be cleverly marketed and bring in another few thousand. That's it! The flat is rented, mostly furnished, and my few thrift shop items are worthless (despite my claim that the kitchen plywood may be original Knoll). There's this computer, which I wouldn't inflict on a dog—not my best purchase, and impossible to get rid of, I suspect.

Despite my occasionally kvetching about being so totally unpropertied, I want to claim here that it was on purpose. It represents a political act/choice, and it is one of the satisfactions I wish to claim at this point. It refers to a frankly youthful and naive point of view, constructed out of Woody Guthrie/Joe Hill songs ("My will is easy to decide / For I have nothing to divide") and a curiously 1960s American Zen version of the vow of chastity, poverty, and obedience—in which obedience was inverted to disobedience, chastity was understood to be of the spirit, and a rider promised that the devotee would neither sit nor sleep above the level of the floor. Implicit in all this was the idea that one wouldn't own property, notably real estate (i.e., New Mexico communes were deeded to "God" or abstract collectives). Credit cards were highly suspect unless they were stolen or intended for nefarious objectives.

Various people attempted to label and articulate this vague hippy leftist economic ethic. I remember "Lord Byron," guru of "The Family" (not Manson's—just) where I lived during 1970 in Taos, lecturing us on the "forward flow of money," which included as a central principle that we do not possess property (lest it possess us), but we only use;

when a thing's utility is exhausted, for the user, the possession is "cut loose." This model has points of contact with what I understand Warlpiri economics—in a simplified ideological gloss, as if one could strip all the complex kin and ritual exchange systems from its practice—to produce. But, as it turned out, the "forward flow of money" in fact required biannual trips to the keno tables at Reno; the last ending in total disaster, but that's another story. Mostly, these public articulations of collective hippy economics in the end totally obscured the actual material bases of the communes, the surplus economy on which they depended—inheritances by the children of Pittsburgh banking and steel families, generous allowances from families in Scarsdale and Great Neck, easily available welfare, and toward the end, fairly shocking mega-drug deals, media sellouts, and other tawdry dealings as the 1960s surplus economy dwindled and daddy took the T-Bird away. Second only to the failure to deal in any intelligent, appreciative way with feminism, this was the great disappointment to many of us as the radical movement of the 1960s turned belly-up and we saw exposed the economic bones which had underwritten all that rhetoric. What could be salvaged, I decided, could only be a personal code of ethics, an attempt, as a matter of pride, to stick to vows made when young and foolish, or at least to be explicitly accountable for any deviations. It seems to me I've come close: I own only the property I've just described. I sleep up off the floor now, but on a futon (how that makes it all right has to do, I'm afraid, with a 1980s marketing strategy figured out by entrepreneurial ex-hippies and cleverly aimed at an ex-hippy market, and is designed to resist any closer analysis). I have two credit cards: one for overseas and one for Australia. These became the only possible way of organizing and accounting for my expenditures, particularly when they were to be claimed as expenses for my job, and I consider the outrageous interests charged justified in my case, because I think of all this as the equivalent of having an accountant. I think I've paid income tax only once, at my father's request so he could claim me as a deduction that year. I can get away with that because always they owe me, given my erratic employment record. This might sound quite mad to most people; in the end, I'm losing money, probably a great deal, by these strategies. I must admit to being quite exhausted by it all, and confess that my new, permanent academic appointment seemed most likely to compromise every one of these principles (except maybe the futon). But these economic logics, or illogics, I think, would not seem too alien or silly to my Warlpiri friends. And I maintain here that the point of intersection which generates these similarities between my vaguely Marxist/Zen/hippy economic idiolect and a hunter-gatherer ideology is this resistance to fixed notions of property ownership which is superseded by ideas of custodianship, utility, of "looking after": a processual model. So, I was very comfortable in my life at Yuendumu, and despite the great and painful distances that separated me from the Warlpiri people, I shared a casualness about things, objects, permanencies, which was the source of whatever familiarity was achieved with both the video-makers and the older painters. In many of the same terms as theirs, I wasn't easily fussed, although this was the result of quite different histories. This is why I suspect the people at Yuendumu will appreciate certain aspects of my coming and going through this material world without difficulty, while admitting other issues, such as uttering my name, may prove less comfortable.

* * *

In this dream, I'm in a seaside resort city, made up of all my childhood seasides—Coney Island, Margate, but mostly Atlantic City in the 1960s. I am staying with my father at one of the old hotels several blocks back from the beach. Between us and the beach lies a seedy amusement park, made up of all my childhood amusement parks, mostly Coney Island which I explored so thoroughly in 1961 with my brother Mark.

Dad and I decide to go for a walk on the beach—perhaps I engineer this as an opportunity to finally tell him. I start down the street but he indicates we have to take a detour around the amusement park. "But this street has direct access; we don't need to go five blocks out of the way," I complain. I am already tiring from the walk. He is adamant. I am about to say, "I'm too weak to go the extra blocks because I'm dying of AIDS." But I can't say that because I haven't told him yet. The horns of this apparent dilemma skewer the dream, a head-throb wakes me to the realization that my fever has returned, which makes me feel defeated. It indicates that this fever episode of the last few days is resolving to a cyclical state, not the improving one I had hoped was indicated. Trying to read the body so that one can use it as text for the construction of a narrative called "diagnosis" too easily becomes an obsessive pastime in my condition—aided especially by the fevered imagination. Very soon, so many things seem to go wrong, so many tests need to be tried to identify these. The detective work of piecing together possible jigsaw puzzles is one thing AIDS patients can do with their time. I turn back to thoughts of my dream, it is the first my erratic sleep patterns have encouraged me to recall in months. But so crudely transparent! Have I no subtler symbology by which to mediate my fear of writing the letter to my father, or no more finely drawn characterization of him than this Lacanian cartoon, insisting that we "take the main way" and avoid "the amusement park"?

Another, and stranger, dream this afternoon had me being cared for in the most intimate and comfortable way by a middle-aged woman, someone like Simone Signoret, but not frightening, not frightening at all. One of my disappointments in life is that gayness finally resolved nothing about my tortured relations toward women. It simply provided a distancing device. Now, my women friends share a kind of spectatorship with me: alongside, we comment on things, but barely face each other.

What was so notable about my dream was the utter casualness and simplicity of the woman's concern for me. She held me, talked to me, and in the end, curled up alongside me as I napped. In fact, as I began my nap in the dream, I began to wake in reality, and felt this woman get up from the bed, and sensed a parting glimpse of only her back going out the hospital door as my bed shrunk back to single size.

What I wake to from these dreams is the infectious diseases ward of the Royal Brisbane Hospital, on the edge of a hill overlooking what I have come to regard as this terrible city, built on a mosquitoed inlet on the tropical east coast of Australia. However, if you want to avoid waking directly next to the generator for an 800-bed hospital, you forego the view and try to be booked into a right-side room which looks across the entry drive to an oddly pleasant colonial house and a niche of tropical plantings. Between these two sides runs a long, crooked corridor—littered with wheeled stainless-steel objects, holding or conveying a bewildering assortment of wrapped things, wrapped to protect their sterility, or used, tainted things, wrapped to prevent contamination.

The marvelous thing about all this, I realize as I wake from my dream, is how this place really is one of those superbly rich sites of contradiction, sort of a Foucauldian holy ground on which multiple lines of discourse converge, like ley lines converge at Stonehenge. A person lying in my bed merely looking around the room and out the window can see great distances, to parliamentary debates on condoms and morals, to histories of Australian asylums, etiquettes, hierarchies, and colonialisms. But what most has me flat on my back here is a discourse of "Tidiness."

* * *

In my experience, "tidy" is a word only used by adults when talking (down) to children. The very first time I heard the word used in adult conversation was early on at Yuendumu where its adult usage was limited to "Tidy Town," a competition sponsored by the Northern Territory government which surveyed burgs great and small throughout the area and awarded prizes to the tidiest. Christian fellows at Yuendumu were apt to take this tragically seriously, believing perhaps that the prize provided another coupon for the great Aussie cargo cult in which somehow they were always missing out. So each March, before the judges were due, James and Muk Muk (if they controlled the council that year) would get the big rocks all painted white again, and one year somebody even bulldozed all the trees in town to make the place tidier. Obviously, in the paternalistic context of black/white dialogue, this usage is admittedly specialized.

But in Brisbane "tidy" is nearly a key term, pivotal in the local lexicon and regional ontology. It operates semantically rather like the more general, Australia-wide term "Fitness." Both describe a state mightily desired, nearly a state of grace within the cultural configuration. Persons both tidy and fit are ideal *Perfect Match* partners. And of course, both terms actually obscure the very principles they claim to promote. Fitness substitutes the appearance of health for health itself, often in a most unhealthy manner. Fit people can grog on all day but not seem sick, lying their steroid-pumped-up bodies out in the sun, working on their skin cancer. Tidiness, we will discover by analogy, does not assure the cleanliness it promises. Instead, it merely obscures dirt; indeed, all natural (and finally historical) processes.

I first encountered the discourses of tidiness upon arriving in Brisbane and looking for a place to live. The real estate agents, having assessed my class and finances (remember, here all renters are suspect and assumed to be dags), decided I must be put into a good, "tidy" place. In a city with some of the most interesting regional architecture in Australia, I found it extraordinary that I was shown nothing but a series of brick motel rooms, utterly characterless, wholly unlivable, but, yes, tidy. Eventually, inquiring after an "untidy" flat, I got myself a cheap, quite spectacular bedsitter directly on the river, with two weeks free rent for tidying it up. But it was when I started hunting for furniture that I discovered true sites of significance in the contradictions of tidiness.

There are thousands of antique shops in Brisbane. A few are large barns (often housing many independent stalls), but most are neighborhood shops, selling a small inventory and maintaining a workshop in the rear. These stores dot intersections throughout the neighborhoods of Brisbane like newsagents or chemists do in other cities, implying a vast specialist network and a broad underground economy.

What goes on in these shops is that old furniture is "restored." Quite simply, this means that every sign of age is stripped from the piece; it is dipped, stripped, sanded, polished, varnished, lacquered and acrylicked. The result is always an ultra-glossy product, as indistinguishable as possible from any new wares on the floor of a Myer's department store. Antique originals are converted into their own reproductions.

In Philadelphia, I worked briefly in this same industry, having grown up near the major antique district. What Brisbane restorers were doing to their goods rendered them absolutely worthless from any calculation I had been exposed to. While there were debates about the degrees of refinishing permissible before the patina, the "age" which gave a work its value, was lost, nothing remotely approaching the wholesale resurfacing standard in Brisbane would ever have been imagined, let alone excused.

I never found any polite way to suggest as much to any Brisbane dealers. For, indeed, it was their labor, far more than the objects, that they were marketing. Objects themselves seemed to have no intrinsic interest (except, curiously, the type of wood used). The miracle, and the value, came from the transformation of something old, banal, untidy, to something seemingly new. Even my most oblique remarks—aimed more at discovering where I might find "unrestored" pieces—offended grievously. My attempt to find the sources of unrestored pieces of course was regarded as a competitive intent, and I got nowhere. Eventually, I found a couple of "second-hand" shops. Fortunately, I didn't have much space to fill.

My remarks about Brisbane are meant to demonstrate more than just my conviction that somehow it was this place that done me in. This rather circuitous meditation on tidiness, for example, is meant to bring me back to my bed at Wattlebrae from which I observe somewhat endless rounds of cleaning, cleaning, cleaning. But early on, I detected that the purpose of all this activity probably was more ritual than rational—that the cleaners were instilling tidiness, not fighting disease. So the story of the flat and the furniture is intended to illustrate how this works. Tidiness is a process which, while avowedly in the service of cleanliness and health, in fact is only interested in obscuring all traces of history, of process, of past users, of the conditions of manufacture (the high high gloss). Tidiness inhabits and defines a "moment," but one outside time, ahistorical, perhaps the ancestral Dreamtime home of all "life styles." It is a perfect bourgeois metaphor. The tidy moment does not recognize process, and so resists deterioration, disease, aging, putrefaction. On this basis, it justifies its association with health and cleanliness and is considered an appropriate discourse to inflict on the diseased, the aging, the putrefying.

Twice a day, the floors of Wattlebrae are waxed to the highest possible gloss. The floors are old and cracked linoleum, and the effect, particularly in the sea-blue floor of my room, is quite attractive. But it seems to me that wax has nothing particular to do with germs. Indeed, the result would be to embed bacteria—to preserve them, wouldn't it? To be fair, the floors are also swabbed down twice a day. But the real dramatic effort is the one spent on polishing, and I am convinced it is a tidy, not a healthy, activity. The issue becomes all the more dramatic if you're actually the one sick and on your back. From the staff's upright point of view, the floors must seem quite impressive, but in bed you barely see them. What you do see is the ceiling, paint cracked, peeling and falling into the water jar, ceiling fan blades edged in dirt and encrusted with insects. Tidiness only applies to the perspective of the fit. An identical example is the fuss to clean all dorsal surfaces in my room each day, including, in particular, the mobile table that fits over my bed for eating and typing. The top is cleaned twice. The underside, with which I actually come in contact, hasn't been swabbed since 1942 as far as I can judge.

The matter is more shocking than just this. The very idea that PWAS are placed in an infectious diseases ward seems to me criminal insanity, or extreme malevolence. I do realize that there is a history to that decision and that it represents a victory compared to other solutions which had been advanced (what? stake us to anthills and pour honey on our heads?), and that many people working here are brave and doing their very best. But AIDS is not an infectious disease: darling, if I had to tell you what I went through to get this, your hair would curl pink! But we *are* terribly susceptible to disease. Indeed, my current stay in Wattlebrae has been extended precisely because my white cell count collapsed in response to an injudicious overuse of antibiotics (to attempt to get through a demanding Sydney weekend). Right now, neither of my immune systems is worth shit, and I'm totally vulnerable. So I share facilities, bathroom, and unsealed rooms with some of the most exotic illnesses in the tropical world. The floors may glow, but often as not, the communal toilet is filthy. I'm terrified to go out of my room into this tidy world.

November 16, 1987

Penny flew up from Canberra. I must have looked pretty awful, and out of it, as I can't remember much. She called the States in an effort to track down and tell my family. She got through to my brother (Dad and Mitzi were off to Portugal this particular week). I had drafted and finally sent a very careful, long letter to Dad a few days earlier, part of my complex strategy of disclosure. When Penny told me what she'd done, I was speechless with anger. I must have been terrifying, precisely because I didn't fly off the handle for the first time ever, but just stood there. Then I saw how frightened she was and found myself trying to reassure her, to repair the damage of that unguarded, incredulous glower.

November 22, 1987

Paul came up from Sydney and spent Wednesday and Thursday chewing off my doctor's ear with inquiries about alternative therapies—vitamin C, Israeli egg yolks, macrobiotics—all the while blowing massive clouds of cigarette smoke at me (even carping about my choosing to have a chocolate dessert with my otherwise health-food dinner). What I need to realize is how terribly worried he must be, likewise Penny, and how both utterly lack experience in this sort of thing. So they imagine there is much that must be done, that they must do, and go blustering about in a touching, but quite unnecessary way, getting things "under control," barely masking their own worry and confusion. I think it testifies to how very calm I am that I sit here watching all this happening, nearly in slow motion (while the actual drama can get very frantic), and mostly worrying about my poor friends' feelings.

We did manage to map out a writing/editing program, which feels like an accomplishment. John had apparently suggested that I be told to relax, that "I'd done enough!" What a delicious thought, one that should be boomed down, Cecil B. De Mille–style, from a Technicolor heaven which parts and isolates me in a pool of light while the deepest British voice available intones, "You have done enough!" This pronouncement, welcome as it is, is not really the point. With the final edit of the monograph [*For a Cultural Future: Francis Jupurrurla Makes TV at Yuendumu*], I consider my "obligations" satisfied. What I've been writing now is in some more indulgent sense just for me, and because if I weren't writing, what would I be doing? Paul was intrigued with the drafts of this diary, and suggested ways that the form could provide a framework for a lot of diverse material, a prospect I find very exciting, even if this stretches the designation "diary," even memoir, rather far. He also set out a reading program for me, which begins with Joe Orton's diaries and includes Defoe and Gide. But the only thing he could find in the hospital bookstore was *The Diary of Anne Frank*, which Paul thought a good idea but I think is so bizarre that, for reasons I can't even fathom, I can barely find strength to lift the book so as to hide it under the pile of clothes on the chair by my bed.

Paul thinks Orton's diary is fabulous because it's so full of action: the author's always ducking into the loo to have it off with somebody. Obviously, my present circumstances offer no similar possibilities for active narrative devices. This is part of the justification for moving around in time, so the diary becomes not merely a static chronological meditation, but a kind of time machine which, while always returning to my present terminal illness, ends up with a more general autobiographical range. I am also warned against too much explicit reflexivity, a principle that I agree to, even as I sit here violating it.

Yesterday, I got a blood transfusion, intended to sort of kick-start my slowly improving constitution and counteract my lethargy. It was a bugger of a day, and I was on my back for eight hours, not the four I'd been promised. By the end, I was very cranky. The needle ached from the beginning and, in all, I felt miserably uncomfortable. Nobody had yet got me the books I wanted, and I was stuck with some Ian Watson sci-fi short stories that really are quite unpleasant, no matter how clever.

But the bloody thing worked, and today I had heaps of energy. Lee took me to the New Farm park kiosk for morning tea, where I was quite horrible in my stage-whispered criticisms of the fat middle-class families which scrambled through, hell-bent on more sugar. Then he dropped me at my flat, and for the first time in weeks, I was wonderfully, deliciously, by myself. I immediately searched for my cache of dirty books, took to bed and jerked off. Then I watched a Deborah Kerr godawful black-and-white war melodrama on TV for the rest of the afternoon. Joe Orton, eat your heart out!

December 1, 1987

Australia celebrates today as the first day of summer, and so strips from the season all ritual, cosmological, indeed sacred meanings which are evoked by the solstices. To begin summer based on the arbitrary, civic calculations of a calendar date (a calendar not especially well tied to the celestial at that—a "one," a "first of") is profane in the extreme. But suitable for Australia, I think, and not merely because it seems such a civic culture. Rather, I have experienced extreme confusion with all seasonal rituals since being down here. Christmas in summer? Harvest in spring? And what of the incomprehensible international dateline: how am I to calculate the exact moment of a full moon and so synchronize with friends who might still be celebrating (last of the Mohippies!) such events in the northern hemisphere? Von Sturmer arrived Wednesday and I threw a big Thanksgiving bash for a (the usual) dozen people Friday night on the rationale that this morning people in the U.S. would be sitting down to their turkeys, arguing that this took precedence over the rule that Thanksgivings are always celebrated on Thursdays. This was admittedly pretty post hoc; I had my own reasons for declaring and defining this celebration, and for using up most of the energy from my blood transfusion spending the day exhausting myself utterly in the kitchen. Absolutely everything worked—the stuffing, the pumpkin pie—and the result was more than a passable offering. I even made a little speech on the extraordinary notion that Australians imagine a national holiday similarly celebrating their collaboration with, and gratitude to (fake as the American example may be), the indigenous people of the continent. Ha!

I just took von S. to the airport. He's been here nearly a week. Why aren't these things more fun and less "work" (in that dreadful, social worker sense of the term). In fact, it's a bit difficult to describe what this visit was to work out, and why it didn't—or perhaps it did. My condition two weeks ago may well have justified inciting panic among my nearest and dearest. Obviously, I cannot fault them for their concern or their consequent actions . . . much. For, of course, from where I sat (or more precisely lay) at that time, subjectively alert, mentally engaged, reasonably coherent, I might have been very sick, or in some grave, inchoate danger, but I didn't think that was death. Which reveals to me, finally, what I fear dying is: it's losing your mind, your marbles, going crazy. Which is why the demented fellow Johnno from the next hospital room so terrifies me. When he wanders into my room, I hide under the covers. But when he rails in the hall, tries to get through the locked door in the corridor, plays up on the way to the shower, I listen with obsessive, horrible interest.

Von S. and I had established that I wasn't on the critical list any more, but there really was never any question that he would/should come up. Probably, I need to examine that assumption more closely. Part of the purpose was, I thought, to assist in the transition home from the hospital. Part was to check firsthand to see how I was doing. Part was what I often bring to my dyads with John: a sense of testing, of examination, of the mental—meaning more than merely the intellectual. This examination consists, it sometimes seems to me, of a challenge, but the object of this challenge is precisely to convert the challenge into a collaboration. Having accomplished this, we can talk, and von S. and I sometimes nearly sprout wings and fly just talking. But it does sometimes seem difficult (for von S. or me, I'm not sure) to get into gear. An introductory ritual seems required, and doesn't always succeed; often it is I who am tired and can't bring the terms into focus. By contrast, Paul and I either click, or we don't, right off, although it can be awfully painful if, having not clicked, we can't disengage either, and have to drag around not clicking for a whole afternoon. At least von S. and I can always seem to disengage gracefully.

Except for this time, which is the first I recall. I think simply having anybody around for a full week would have gotten to me. John was exemplary in this respect, repeatedly checking exactly this point with me. But I did really appreciate his company. I was caught in a bind which, as so often happens with me (it's from the mother's side), expresses itself in whinging/nagging. Little things, decidedly, purposely. My immortal soul is at risk, the Queensland government is collapsing, 150 die in a plane wreck off Mauritius, and I'm having a go at John about putting the iron frying pan in water, or forgetting to have the plumber stop the laundry room leak. The strategy, which almost always works, at least on people of insight and good will, soon has John at the breaking point, at which he entitles himself to a single mean word—perhaps less, only an implied criticism, ideally not of my behavior except with respect to how I am treating him. The official method has me now appearing to sulk for some time, while actually worrying my minor wound into a full-scale mortal stroke, and preparing an utterly devastating attack, aimed at the most vulnerable area of the other that my most intimate recollections and obsessive intellect can identify. Then whack!, off with preferably some organ with profound sexual and personal significance, probably in a Lacanian calculation. The advantage of this procedure is, of course, that if you don't make a clean first swipe of it, you get to hack, hack, hack, ever so painfully until all players in this tawdry domestic are drowning in blood and familial guilt.

Obviously, these tendencies must be resisted. And I congratulate myself in the quasi-privacy offered here, for not destroying my relationship with John by recasting us in a drama, which, as I say, was one of Mama's cruelest legacies. Part of this is calculation, a calculation I am surprised my mother apparently failed to make until perhaps her very end—which is that, if one is to be required to develop dependent relationships, and rely on others, wouldn't one prefer to choose who should do this for you? And I suppose, in most instances, those friends, people whose company, ethics, and conversation you enjoy, are to be preferred. In fact, these questions go much more deeply to the heart of the matter than I intended, and to my difficulties with John . . . and Paul and Penny, my father and siblings, perhaps the whole of my real and potential social matrix, which now I find myself reexamining, and at the grossest level, in terms of suitability for the role of personal butler, nurse, secretary, companion, cook, etc. John is too sloppy, but Paul is too fussy; Pen gets upset too easily, and so on. Utterly impossible criteria and quite unfair, because, if nothing else, these were not the terms on which our friendships were based or grew. And yet, I do fantasize about some assistance, some increased comfort, something personified, as romance was once personified in the image of the Lover.

December 3, 1987

Liz flew in from Sydney. How do I avoid turning these accounts of visits into grading exercises? Liz gets a B+, John a C, and so forth. And how do we grade the assessor? Still, I thought Liz did quite well, and I really did appreciate her company, her talk, and her offers of help, even if I didn't so much show it. Once, I went quite off the handle and yelled at her, so maybe she thinks she screwed up, when in fact I thought her quite sensitive.

What Liz did was scan the situation, figure out what she could do (rather than any more abstracted and undelimited notion such as "what needs to be done"). She offered to approach the Minister for Immigration and attempt to get me residence through his direct intervention. I thought this very clever of her: not just in case she might pull it off, but because indeed this would be the only means of providing some security for me and reducing my anxiety about being tossed out (where? into the gutter? the sea?) at any moment by the forces of the state. So it would be the best possible Christmas present. Considering how naive other offers (to "care" for me) have proved to be, I am really touched by Liz's good sense here.

December 6, 1987

The History and Film Conference at the University of Queensland: I was supposed to give a paper, then I wasn't; I was on the program, then off. I couldn't imagine what was going on. Stuart, in his role as a convener, seemed to wish some uncharacteristic alignment between text and life, and kept revising the program entry announcing my paper presumably on the basis of current hospital reports. When finally Lee brought the printed program over Friday night (not Wednesday, as Stuart—whose answering machine I'd talked to a dozen times since then—had promised), my name was crudely penned in on this particular copy. I felt horribly insulted and proceeded to bitch to everyone within range.

The problem, of course, is that I had to hear myself as well, and two things struck me: first, that I'd always been on the other end of these prima donna conference performances (an academic who isn't quite first-rate discovers this suddenly in the midst of a conference and begins to demand the prerogatives of a major luminary to everybody's profound embarrassment). And second, that I had better get more careful right quick about alienating the decreasing number of allies who may be willing to help me in my hour of dependency—except both my tendency and, furthermore, my politics insist that this is precisely the moment one becomes most insistent, most insanely principled, even childishly stubborn. But this is constrained by the simultaneous fear that my rationality is becoming strained (such a delicate, indeed, Queensland way to put it!), that my mind is not able to manage the subtleties of calculation and perception required of such strategies. I still have no clear idea of what happened with/to John, and even I am not especially convinced by these post hoc accounts which rationalize the last week's visits, and things are taking on somewhat too plastic dimensions, recalled mythically mostly. Or, more simply, my fever's up again.

I recanted and went to the conference, reading from the monograph galleys, and giving a passable performance to the seven or eight people clever enough to find out about it and come. Not a major event from any angle, but I handled myself, and the questions, reasonably well, as I feel it has become essential to do. H—— C—— was there, and took me aside for a chat, although it is generally reckoned he is rather too much of a schmo to get anywhere. How does Tom O'R. manage it then? In introducing me, Tom O'Regan spent some time trying to apologize for his embarrassingly fulsome public praise at the Australian Screen Studies Association Conference last year, and stepped right smack in the same paddy of poo again!

Liz called and started to tell me why Mick Young [the Minister for Immigration] wasn't allowed to let me stay in the country unless I had a wife/lover here. Compassion is restricted to pair bonds. There seems no solution. But in the service of being an accurate reporter and helpful friend, she started from the beginning and was proceeding to give me the entire sequence of endless bureaucratic illogic. I had to get her off the phone, brutally, finally because listening to that shit again was driving me mad. I said Liz, stop it, that's what made me sick in the first place: these endless dissertations on why, because I reject nationalism, and the nuclear family (for my own practice, at least), I have no rights, no rights at all . . . and I may die in a way which I, but maybe only I, believe has elements of murder. I have no focus for this anger. My fever logged in at 39 degrees by the time I got off the phone, after weeks of normal readings.

December 9, 1987

Two teeth out yesterday. EEG this A.M. Things remain more medicalized than they were supposed to. I go to the hospital daily, as other people go to a job. Finally had a chat to Dr. K. about all that, and he gave me a day off (tomorrow). I won't have to report in at all, unless, of course, my fever flares up again as it's been threatening to do. I'm getting quite testy about getting poked at for no evident result. But the failure to construct a believable medical diagnosis/narrative is itself grounds for some concern. Essentially, I seem to have just about everything you could have. I will endure, or not, on the basis of my general constitution and my capacity to keep my immune system up. That's all.

While I do my inhaler, I read Steegmuller's Cocteau biography. At first I read Orton's diary. (Hated his attempts to elevate class traitorship to . . . what, art? Sleazy, but not in the prudish, prurient way implied.) I thought it terrible, to be trapped in Orton's world of abject self-deception, utterly lacking the ironization that Fassbinder, say, gives to the same theme in the *Desire*. But, for Orton, this is no theme. He really believed he was gorgeous. Cocteau proves a more pleasant world to escape to, providing even amusing resonances (my inhaler = Jean's opium). What is it we envy today about such worlds (the locales of various bohemias, mostly New York or Paris, but sometimes Tangiers, Black Mountain, Bloomsbury, etc.)? Presumably, it is the assurance of creative community, preferably one which will be acknowledged, and the delicious mise-en-scènes generated at such sites. But, in the case of the Steegmuller, I think something is missing from his account of this, and his account of Cocteau. It is the profound moral imperatives and ethical calculations that ultimately do drive great gay queens throughout this century (and the last, as far as it can be determined). Steegmuller's accounting is nearly all gossip; it operates within the web of gossip, which gives equal weight to all news. When in fact what Cocteau is involved in is a formation and application of discriminations: attributions of value, which is indisputably an onerous responsibility always pivoting on the capacity not merely for desire, but even more for denial, in the service of something—Cocteau would likely identify it as the sublime—which, in any case, has quite different, and more difficult, objects than Steegmuller's account implies. It is the only possible (but altogether sufficient) justification for wearing Chanel black and a single string of pearls. It is the only note that can be struck when you lean against the piano, to sing. . . .

December 12, 1987

Discharged from the hospital to satisfy some inscrutable bureaucratic requirement (to avoid being listed as a chronic medical dependent, or something). Buranda Labor Club Christmas party in Annerley. The club is an apparently Lee-generated circle; on some nights it masquerades as the Fanny Street Saturday Night Gender-Bender Soiree, it shows up at Stuart's in Highgate Hill as the Weekend Punkers Dance Groupies, and we marched in the May Day parade as the Contra-Trotsky / Contra-Libertarian / Post-Althusserian / Labor-Not-So-Left (Any More). But it's the same dozen or so people each time. Not even a group I'm particularly wild about, or have great times with. But this is Brisbane, and I suppose we all make do.

I do get to wondering about how I got to this dreadful place, and why I'm stuck here, and as long as I am here, what on earth I'm going to do. I've never thought of my illness as a punishment. But that's exactly how I think of Brisbane. I am so minimally connected here. I have only two local friends to speak of (which is not to say only two people are nice to me, but rather that I've only discovered Stuart and Lee to talk to). That's a pretty thin anchor to a place. And as I survey the various gestures and attempts to set up some kinds of support which I'm told will be (already are) necessary for me to live outside of hospital, it's clear that I will have difficulty assembling even the minimal personnel to be effective or reliable. The Queensland AIDS Council [QuAC] itself seems terminally hopeless—caught up in that characteristic Australian cult which puts all energy into protocol/politics and imagines that acts and actions will magically result from correct ideological thought.

So I imagine, despite all the flurry of apparent activity and kind intentions, I need to face up to the fact that I remain comparatively alone in all this, with a good deal of distant backup, but nothing to get me through the night. And that at some point early-to-mid next year, I'll have to depart Brisbane, for one reason or another, one way or another.

December 15, 1987

Ruined, ruined, what a bugger of a day! Everything was going to get done at once: QuAC cleaner, and carpet people, installing the ceiling fan. And Lee, dear Lee, was to coordinate all this, and that was crucial, because as you know, dear diary, I cannot deal with Brisbane people directly without getting into horrible fights.

Well, Lee missed our Saturday lunch, without notice, so I never did get briefed on what would happen Monday, and finally Monday morning I called him, and he said he was on his way over. He got here after the QuAC cleaner (which already had me terrified, simply because dealing with strangers is far too difficult right now). The carpet cleaners came not at noon, but about 10:30 A.M., which kind of confused things, and proceeded to spray an unbearable scent around. Of course! That's what this carpet cleaning is about, and why only in Brisbane are references to it made in one's lease. It's not about cleaning at all. It's about perfuming, called "deodorizing"; again, a variant of the discourses of tidiness. And again, this false cleanliness risks making me sick. I fled the flat, and went shopping. When I returned, 40 minutes later, Lee had already left. The stench was unbearable, so I stood on the back steps and talked to the QuAC fellow. The carpet steamers had apparently handed him some cock-and-bull story about the carpet being an old one, with no underlay (bull! it's a new one with no underlay—admittedly a cheap, tricky solution to carpeting), which was presumably to cover their failure to get the place very clean. But I discovered when I returned three or four hours later (hoping the smell had gone, knowing it never would, amazed that the carpet was still wet despite the promise of "one hour dry") that they had rent two huge, intersecting slashes in the carpet, certain to cost me my security deposit, not to mention the increase in ugliness and disorder I would have to live in/with. Meanwhile, all the furniture had been moved, and many books, files, and implements from my study as well, so that I was left alone in this stinky flat, with an entire furniture-moving project on my hands before I could even get into the bathroom or use my desk! This was the result of all this assistance on our truly helpful day. I am in the subbasement of despair. I sat up all night, inhaling this unbearably cheap, poisonous scent, cursing Lee, but even more painfully aware that there was no point complaining to him, or anybody for that matter. I could simply move back into the hospital, get on a plane for Boston, or pray I don't get any more ill and helpless than I am now.

December 17, 1987

Have been going into school, catching up on correspondence mostly. Also, it gets me out of bed. I really am getting bored in a way I think Brisbane either causes, or at least cannot solve. It is that hideously weird limbo time of year; everybody is leaving town, rather like air escaping from a whoopee cushion. Stuart and Jo headed down to Sydney. Lee's staying. David McC. and Merlin visited tonight; when Mary gets here we can all socialize together . . . the last inhabitants of Brisbane. And of course, all this is tied up with familialities. One either is or isn't going home for Christmas. "Isn't" seems to require as much engaged confrontation with family as "is." I wish I could go over to Philly and Boston for a two-week visit without Immigration barring my return.

Melissa is coming December 29, so I will have the odd, but welcome experience of blood kin again. What an extraordinary burden to put on a young woman's shoulders: to make the first visit to the dying uncle —to map the lie of the land. One of Melissa's most attractive traits is exactly this remarkable sense of being a responsible sort, a rarity which endears us all to her all the more. It will be interesting to see what gaps we can bridge and which distances we enforce during this week or so of a sustained encounter of mutual admiration, but comparative mystery.

Phone has been ringing off the wall. I had no idea I knew so many people, had so many people to talk to. Dad called last night (Dr. K. was here and got a chat in), David Nash called just now. In talking to David, I realized almost everybody we knew in common (Françoise, Marcia, Chris and Lee, Nash and Simpson, Toyne, Laughren) had called or written in the last week. I am still quite breathtaken by these shows of support, no less because of the apparent contrast to the very reserved conduct which governed most of these relationships all these years. There is a curious process of accounting going on, one which certainly cheers me up, even if it is occasioned by somewhat morbid circumstances.

December 19, 1987

Went into hospital for tests noon yesterday, out noon today. If you aren't really ill, it becomes clear how unutterably boring hospitals really are. Yankee Johnno, who had been so demented and violent, came in to chat (at Dr. R.'s suggestion). Truly amazing. (Dr. D. had said, incredulously, "It's just like talking to your accountant"—perhaps too much so, as he seems now rather average.) Remarkably, he didn't find out he had AIDS until a week or two ago. Out of nowhere, he just went mad, and then was unable to make sense of (or remember) anything he might have been told during the period of dementia.

All this is encouraging, inasmuch as I'm in for tests to see if my brain is shrinking, and this is the source of my occasional headaches. A most unpleasant thought. For better or worse, I currently have no certain diagnosis of opportunistic diseases except KS—which implies a rather positive prognosis. My chest isn't reacting the way it should for PCP, and there's no clear evidence of anything else, just a lot of maybe's. So, Dr. R. is on a fishing expedition, which is okay with me if it doesn't hurt. Martin called today and we swapped symptoms for an hour. I claimed more faith in official medical research on AIDS (or maybe just a lot less in "alternatives") than I would have expected.

Hospital, other than boring, was okay. Only one nurse flew off the handle (when I pointed out she was 45 minutes late with my AZT medication, and I got one of the more dramatic "don't blame me" speeches of the week). But then . . . ! I forgot my pills, and called up the ward to see if they could get them sent. I had a run-in with the switch who put me through to "enquiries" and who, when I got insistent, kept putting me on hold (to some simpering Muzak), and then breaking in to ask if I was "ready to talk" and then putting me back on hold. Within 45 seconds, I was totally psychotic. I hung up, became DOCTOR Michaels, called and complained to the switch supervisor, and got through to Wattlebrae, who said they'd put my pills in a cab and send them home. Only, the cabbie couldn't read the number on the door and called the hospital back, in the end charging me ten dollars. I screamed vile obscenities at him, called his supervisor and complained too, and was offered a bureaucratic procedure to follow for complaints (are they mad?). I said I just wouldn't use their service again, and I'd advise the hospital of how they exploited a terminal cancer patient in the delivery of his medicine just days before Christmas! I had myself in tears.

Lee came over to return my car. Lee, I said, I feel like they can smell me now, like an injured member of the pack. . . . And they go for me, the sons of bitches, they go for the throat!

December 20, 1987

Read through Stewart Brand's *The Media Lab*. The future he claims they're "inventing" at MIT seems pretty old and awful: all masculinist, techno-driven, socially ignorant and veddy, veddy elite. Caused me to question what the *Whole Earth Catalogue* was really about, and again, who paid for hippydom. Jerry Wiesner was spot-on to credit Brand with delivering up the alternate culture to computerland (it could have gone either way, he notes).

December 24, 1987

Hyperhumbug. Terrible Monday came and went. The electricians put in the ceiling fan: estimate $30; bill $158. A small gland in the pit of my stomach releases a previously unknown but now familiar hormone into my system. My hemoglobin drops another quarter point. T-cells face the firing squad. All my lesions buzz, hum, light up, and claim another millimeter of flesh. I try desperately to understand everything, in relation to me and everything else, to gauge my own paranoia, which, of course, is that paranoia's favorite holiday delicacy. Dr. K. says my brain isn't shrinking at all, no sign of anything. The newspaper reports that 65 percent of HIV carriers (symptomatic or not) exhibit signs of dementia.

Tuesday, off to school (I am apparently the only faculty member who feels required to make these regular appearances any more) for lunch with Athol. He's making a visible effort to engage me, to get to know me, perhaps become friends. I, in return, talk too much, which has become a recurrent problem whenever I have so few opportunities for talk, like now.

The dreaded letter from the Immigration Department was in my box, and I called "my" lawyer, who didn't seem to have a clue. The truly awful part, as I explained to Athol who was in my office at the time, is that I am at least as concerned about being ripped off by the electricians and what to do about the carpet cleaners' stuff-up as the fact that I'm going to be deported in 30 days. Everything now has equal weight, equivalent agro—which, I think, is the surest mechanism of pathological thinking. On the phone to Liz, who zooms to some sort of rescue. She's been on to the Minister again, and the Gay Immigration Task Force person (and lets me in on some of the personal relations that connect these folks and us and everybody else—I'll never adjust to the scale of Australian demography). Nobody can tell me whether to respond to the letter or risk ignoring it. But Liz's industry, connections, and concern are reassuring.

I've gotten a lot of mail, enough to decorate the mantelpiece even, and the phone has kept going until a few days ago. But now, as the holiday really clamps its jaws down on sultry Brisbane, my inevitable isolation and ennui set in. Fine with me, except my energy seems to go with it. For one who responds to honest questions about what I'm doing for Christmas by singing a chorus of Hatikvah and asking if that isn't the day the bread doesn't get delivered, I can hardly complain of a lack of invitations. But all I really want to do is watch telly, except, this is the weirdest part, telly has gone on holiday too. Now, to an American this is inconceivable, and so I'm slammed back to that critical distance—discourses of antipodean alterity—that I wanted to collapse, avoid, escape. The amount of U.S. import seems especially high right now, and the prospect of escaping home through the tube seems reasonable. But no. One is instead overwhelmed by the "différend," not the "simulacrum." And the fact that Australians have no idea: they think they're watching the same TV as the Yanks. . . . They imagine they're becoming Yanks. And you're not allowed to tell them that they're actually becoming something much more like Filipinos.

In the States (if memory serves) holiday times are recognized as times of stress and danger, so that TV is required to perform its most ritualized, integrating, and metronomic functions. Programs and scheduling become ultra-predictable. Jane Pauley has to take her holiday some other time. Millions of dislocated citizens depend on the normal, usual program schedule, especially those "bracketing" shows (news, current affairs), to function; likewise with major serials. To prevent millions from going totally off and grabbing the shotguns and potshotting in the street, TV has a responsibility to demonstrate its reliability. In Australia, it's the opposite, partly because "We're all just workers here, mate!", and the distance between TV personality and audience member is calculated very differently; the social architecture of the electronic proscenium is utterly different—a world in which everybody hibernates for two months of summer. TV is reduced to old documentaries from South Africa, *Beverly Hillbillies* reruns (I get up early for these), and whatever else is at hand.

Amazingly, *Dallas* showed up again, picking up where it dropped off ten months ago, and catching up double-time by being aired as two-hour "specials." No wonder it succeeded here only briefly. It never was aired in its proper rhythm, never allowed its metronomic function, never connected to time on the other side of the tube as it is in the States. Instead, it was aired in contexts based on BBC schedules which effectively reasserted critical distances and subjected its audience to a Brechtian regard; it's a wonder it has any fans here at all!

December 25, 1987

I may be guilty of the ultimate Oz faux pas. I have done my laundry on a holiday. When I went to hang it out, I discovered the small communal yard occupied by set table, chairs, even a paper pineapple centerpiece. Some unconscious Australian cultural rule number 532 must say, "The Hills Hoist in the barbecue area must be vacated on major festival days." Dumb me! Now, my rules say, "If you're planning to appropriate unilaterally a communally owned space, you advise other possible users in advance." Due to these differences in cultural content, we are now on Australian rule number two: "Never voice complaints to those you think responsible." My neighbors seem to be glaring at me. Just glaring. I suspect there's a lot of glaring around Brisbane this time of year.

December 27, 1987

Irony for the week (day? minute? second?): the less that's going on, the more time I have to spend diary writing, and, ipso facto, the less there is to write . . . or rather, write about. My faithfulness as a correspondent this week proves this. I've felt locked in. Everybody who can has apparently fled Brisbane, so no visits, no visitors. Everything's closed, of course. I've got some cranky chest-and-head condition I'm trying to fight back by taking it easy rather than dosing it with antibiotics. It makes me nervous about undertaking anything more ambitious than a trip to the shops. It's hot and muggy, and the awful glare of this sun triggers a headache.

I've spent a good deal of time (and money, I think) on the phone: Liz, Paul, John, and even Gavin H. called on Christmas Day. These are actually "phone visits" of a type I've never indulged in so shamelessly before. Their object is mere sociability, except Liz's, who's still trying to solve the Immigration Department problem, and Paul's, who spends some time on texts. But mostly I feel I should have my hair up in curlers, be poured into capri pants and tiny halter top (with pink rhinestone poodle belt), and take these calls lying upside down on a split-level staircase with black curlicue wrought-iron railing.

I've been watching a great deal of telly. Mostly old Ginger Rogers movies (*Forever Female*, this arvo). And reading the Frank Moorhouse book *(The Everlasting Secret Family)* that Stuart gave me for Christmas. (Is Moorhouse gay? To me, *Family* reads like a straight fantasy of gayness. But my rules predict that for a heterosexually defined male to engage so boldly in such detailed speculation propels him across the border somehow, so he becomes. . . . On the other hand, Australia certainly must offer idiosyncratic homosexualities I can barely imagine: Altman's surely is one.)

In the midst of the odd and offhanded TV schedule, ABC is showing *The Singing Detective*, which must be the most obsessive depiction of desire ever aired as a serial (excepting, perhaps, *My Mother The Car*). And I was locked-in totally the first airing three weeks ago, not only for the uncanny resonances with my own situation (psoriasis, hospital, the immobilization of creativity), but because it was so unlikely on television. Utterly painful, evoking—especially in its presentation of sexuality—the term "adult" as a classification of media long past when such terms seemed useful. How, then, could it claim any audience at all? Who, and how many viewers would subject themselves to this? (How many fellow sufferers are out there?, I beg to ask as a viewer; which is the same question, I think, that the main character asks all the way through, in a manner so reflexive that this may prove the clue to the whole transgeneric mystery.) And, add to this a fully postmodern deconstructed polynarrative justified by reference to detectivisms (generously cited in multiple forms: noir, investigative, literary, etc.).

Of course, there have been no reviews of this extraordinary series, at least none that come to my attention in Brisbane, and no particular notice of its extraordinary oddness at all. So that when I had trouble remembering what night it was on, and couldn't find it in the schedule (a needle that mightn't be in the haystack in the first place), I missed the second episode. But I found tonight's, the third. This furthers the fragmentation of my experience of the narrative, and yet I enjoy and understand something sufficiently to follow it.

Why can't I accomplish the same damn effect with this bloody journal? I read through most of it last night: the textual moves I made from other journals, the juxtapositions of time and place, etc., and the effect isn't riveting at all. (Hence, they have subsequently been removed.) It seems to me merely confusing: I leave nothing generic for the reader to hang on to. Worse, my own posthumous editorial voice keeps resurrecting from a cheaply ironized gallows (as I'm doing now) to confound utterly the cacophony of voices I employ throughout. Hoping the effect will be art is even more arrogant than hoping the effect will be sense.

December 28, 1987

What I do mostly is lie in bed and compose letters of complaint and revenge, intended to repay the shits who are trying to kill me. Like:

Dear Scott

I'm sorry to hear your real estate business is going broke. That, at least, is the only possible interpretation I can give to your recent theft of my security deposit for the Pixley Street flat. Charging for cleaning is illegal, and outrageous, considering the improvement in the place (even so, I couldn't get it up to livable standards and had to move for health reasons despite hundreds of my own dollars spent on decorating and repairs). Charging for a locksmith is utterly unjustified. You might as well have charged the catering bill for your office Christmas party (indeed, maybe you did just that).

I was appreciative of your apparent sincerity during my residence; how as another new Brisbaner, you also acknowledged astonishment of how mercenary a place it was, and how easy it was to get ripped off. I trusted that you were steering me in a better direction. What a good laugh you must be having now as you count and recount the $120 you've robbed me of, probably now converted to 20¢ pieces so as to savor your cheap victory better.

Of course, I realize how inconvenient it must have been for you that I took critically ill and was taken to hospital for a month just as I was moving out. But even with my last breath I paid my bills, arranged for a new tenant, and thought I was due some consideration, as I was considerate of you. Ha! Well, matey, you seem to have adjusted to your new environment better than me, and are likely now to be nickel-and-diming your way to the top in true Queensland style. My lawyer hates handling these petty claims, but when he gets back from holiday I'll ask him to do everything he can to have you thrown in prison where you belong.

Yours sincerely, etc.

Gary, you asshole, M——

Because you kept the video recorder, after Lee told you to return it, and after I pleaded with you to hand it over, several things have happened you should know about and think on. You know I had about 20 hours of tape that had to be logged as part of my attempt to cover a problem that arose between the Aborigines I work with and the Powerhouse Museum. I did try dragging myself out of bed and going to school, but all the studios were closed and there were no video facilities available. Even so, the difference between logging the 20 hours at home and trying to do it on campus means a great deal to my health and limited energy.

Nevertheless, the result has been that I've had to cancel my trip to Sydney (the one holiday I'd hoped for, even if a working one) because I don't have the tapes done. The project, which was important to the Aborigines and important to the Museum (on the argument that it was important to the couple of million people who would have seen it), is jeopardized. And the pressure on me, the fucking stress of all this, and the disappointment takes another toll. I thought you would have taken these things into consideration, at least after I had the demeaning experience of having to spell them out to you, directly and through Lee, then Grahame. As lefties and faggots, I imagined we shared some priorities and terms of debate. Wrong again!

You know I think I've been getting shit all around since I've gotten to Queensland, that I just can't deal with the greed, the rip-offs, the abject self-interest that I found here. I was assured, however, there were exceptions—good people, politically motivated, committed collectively—among whom I might find some friendship and relief. You were promoted as one of these more honest, more concerned people.

So, I ignored the ghastly bourgeois colognes you douse yourself with. I even tried to ignore the horribly insulting infantile sexual come-ons you employed (if that's what they were supposed to be), which embarrassed me personally and raised grave doubts about your interpersonal politics. Because I hardly expected you to turn out to be one of the shits . . . one of the people whose actions (wittingly, or merely through their own selfish egotism) make me ill and whom I must resist at cost of my life.

Hope you had a good holiday and enjoyed all your rent-a-videos right through. Don't ever talk to me, and, more to the point, stay far, far out of my way. Of course, I will not send you this letter. But I shall include it in my diaries and hope that my editors include it in the posthumous publication so that you will be inscribed forever in shame and political disgrace.

Yours, etc.

Dear Turbo Steam Electronic Carpet Cleaning Company

We all make mistakes: it's no crime to admit it. For example, I made a mistake responding to the circular you left in my mailbox, and calling you in to clean my carpets. But $30 seemed so reasonable a rate.

You made a mistake not only by somehow slicing through the middle of my living room carpet in three long lines by some malfunction of your equipment. This is an understandable mistake; I assume anybody in the business would have insurance or some procedure for handling such occasional problems. But you made a bigger mistake in lying about it; inventing a cock-and-bull story about the carpet being old (it isn't) and overly worn (it's not) and falling apart at a glance (bullshit!), and then implying that it didn't even happen.

I am, as a result, likely to lose my $500 security deposit on the apartment (I have no doubt my humanitarian landlord will want at least a full new carpet installed). So, it was a very expensive cleaning job. As you well know, the legal replies open to me are limited. It would cost more to seek satisfaction than I could gain, a fact all you shonky penny-ante predators depend on. So I will take the Richard Nixon payback pledge and curse you with it. Until hell freezes over, I will periodically take whatever opportunity I have to make your life miserable, by mail, by phone, by press—whatever opportunity. Rest assured: you'll be hearing from me.

Forever Yours, etc.

December 29, 1987

Niece Melissa got in from Philadelphia today. I picked her up at the airport, amazed that she arrived when scheduled. I didn't think anything was working, or still scheduled. As a result, I didn't really expect her, wasn't overly uptight and am quite looking forward to enjoying the visit.

On the way out of the parking lot, another Aussie queue jam, and me with no idea what to do. Still, the family-stuffed panel van seemed justified by no imaginable etiquette to claim the space in front of me. Fortunately, my horn is off. I pulled instead a fairly usual Yankee/Philly (black?) routine, overdramatizing a mime of politeness, indicating "Please . . . you first" with a broad sarcastic wave.

The guy stopped, rolled down his window, and asked in all apparent sincerity, "Are you crazy?" I was shattered, had no reply, was mortified in front of Melissa, and wondered whether I should try and conceal my growing pathological bitterness, realizing it was already too late. I wondered how much I would look like my monster mother at her horrible worst in that last decade of her spoiled, indulgent life.

December 31, 1987

New Year's Eve. I was going to have a small group over, mostly Mary L., but she called to say brother Pat was hosting a party and why didn't we come to that. Not a moment too soon (although I had hurt feelings a bit, not to play host), because I felt I was talking Melissa's ear off and she desperately needed to see/meet someone else. Stuart called, having just gotten back from Sydney, and invited us over on the way.

I'd been feeling ratshit. Yesterday, drove Melissa to see the Tall Ships (a few bizarre things that might be masts and sails floating above a bleak, endless, poisonous industrial landscape north of Wynnum) and then to the Gold Coast for a swim. So much voluptuous flesh, such unwelcome thoughts, and me, ashamed and cowering, despite how much I wanted to jump in the cleansing water, and how very few people there were on the spit that perfect morning. Melissa got sunburnt, I lapsed into fever again. Spent today in bed. Got up, and dressed flash at 9 P.M. for dinner and parties. Made it till 2:20 A.M. okay.

Just as well that Melissa see this indescribable contradiction between illness and wellness which appears to alternate in PWAS. In fact, I doubt we are ever quite so well as we appear, but there is good purpose to these public performances.

Pat's party was good. Felt chatty, and comfortable. Lot of Koories there. Jeannie Bell kissed me at midnight, which did touch me. I take it that the disclosure of my condition is now nearly universal. But maybe not, maybe only the connected people, friends, associates; the more general and possibly more hostile public is yet to log in. Chatted a lot to Nancy from the honors course, who was worried, and supportive, and a very pleasant, unassuming lit. lecturer from the University of Queensland who surely thought me a raving asshole. Still, all this does represent a beginning of resurfacing from the terrible journey to Hades of this holiday season, experienced mostly as talk, as the renewed opportunity for conversation and the possibility that my recent pathology is just what you'd expect from somebody who's spent the last few weeks mostly talking to himself.

January 1, 1988

Australia celebrates the New Year and the start of the Bicentenary with a bizarre four-hour telecast "linking up" hundreds of different sites, intending an electronic community, bridging finally the tyranny of distance. Very McLuhan, very New York video freaks, circa 1970. The subject of this extravaganza is nearly no more than the medium itself; so little content emerges, which seems to say something about the Bicentenary and Australian cultural history. But if the telecast doesn't exactly prove McLuhan wrong (the message as the medium can itself be vacant, or at least tedious—we had assumed in the 1970s that such networks would be riveting, if only we could get access to the machinery), it again raises some serious questions: what persisted was narrative, character, and nationalism. Conceptual and process art did not conquer the world.

January 5, 1988

I have sent Melissa off for a day in Sydney before she returns to the States. It's the least she deserves. I think she's very brave to accept the role of emissary for the whole family (such as it is) to go halfway around the world to test the waters regarding faggot uncle dying of fatal disease in unknown land. I was going to send her to John, or Paul, or Liz, but Stuart pointed out (guilelessly), "They're all psychopaths!" So we sent her off to Ross, who's more fun, more her age, and probably won't become utterly consumed by bitterness for another five or even ten years.

I don't feel entirely comfortable reporting my conversations with Melissa. I, of course, did most of the talking, which she encouraged every time I pulled back. She thought me wonderfully "blunt"; I gather that Jill, Dad and everybody still strategize their conversations with her. . . . And there might be a point, she seems sensitive and perhaps might hurt easily, only I don't know how to go about calculating these sorts of things. So I was blunt. And sometimes I detected tears on her cheeks, and, Oh Lord, women crying again!

There was a certain amount of gossip and family intrigue it was fun to get at: What about my new stepmother? Did Jill and Mark fight over what to do about me? And especially, what is Dad up to? Indeed, I remain curious about Jill's feminist reading of my father's paternalism, and wonder how this new marriage fits in. Moreover, I'm somewhat distraught that Dad is treating me so adultly, so noninterventionist. Can't anybody see that I don't have a clue how to handle all this? Oh well, I'm sure nobody else does either. There was also a good deal I needed to cover with respect to mad mother and her final scenes. I gather that these were easier for Melissa because she could accept that Mom was a mess, and proceed from there. I (and maybe my siblings) kept fighting that.

If my family is to take any major responsibility for my care—i.e., if I return to the States—we will have to invent that family.

January 15, 1988

Five days in Sydney. I'm completely buggered. Paul's new boyfriend was sick; he called and sensibly suggested I not stay there until the situation was more clear. Called John (whose silence the last few weeks, after not arriving after Christmas, I thought very odd), and had him book me into the Manhattan. It turned out they'd doubled their prices again, painted everything pink and gray, and completed the task of making a modest, comfortable country-style hotel utterly uninhabitable. After two days (spent mostly video editing at Metro TV—also frustrating as the Powerhouse people haven't a clue what they want) of sweltering in a room without even a sink and five degrees hotter than outside, and noisy as hell, I checked out and took to the streets.

Liz took me in, or rather I forced myself on her. I could indulge not a single additional minute feeling sorry for myself. (Where are all these people who were meant to be taking care of me? I didn't feel very good, or strong.) She fussed and fussed, concerned that her guest room was too moldy and wet. So great, I should sleep on the street?

In the middle of the night, I had a very noisy dream that scared the shit out of Liz. Oddly, I recall making the noises. Perhaps I was trying to wake myself up from a nightmare. My cries went on for over ten minutes, Liz says. But what I remember was having discovered a "generative grammar of dream." What I imagined myself doing as I woke (I was very close to the surface when Liz finally came in) was stringing together the "phonemes of dream." But this was a totally structural exercise; my cries, in my explanation, precisely had no meaning. My first words were thus an apology to Liz. I realized I scared her with what I considered merely a form of play.

Next two days spent at Paul's. Boyfriend (I approve) recovered. Paul absolutely drove me through two days of editing: monograph galleys, and then *Art & Text* essay draft ["Bad Aboriginal Art"]. We both started to get bitchy toward the end; me, I thought, with somewhat more justification. How dare he accuse me of being lazy with my references (after I was commanded to do just that to save energy!). And how dare he tell me that Paul Taylor says nobody in New York reads these Aboriginal pieces anyway! Fortunately, by the time it came to that, John was there to fight some of the battle for me. I was completely buggered.

What is this, anyway? This was supposed to be my vacation—just a little bit of work, and time to shop, see movies, friends. No movies, no shopping, just friends chaining me to their various grindstones. This is very odd. Only a week or so ago I was an invalid. Now they've got the whip out again. Obviously, all indulgences are terribly short-lived, while the disease drags on.

And, in fact, I suspect I am at the end of my last transfusion, turning paler and paler, and moving slower . . . and slower. . . . (Funny, you can convey that phonically, or denote it with script, a bit with type, but not at all with the computer.)

January 16, 1988

I've come back from a meeting with my Dean. It's a great idea to place sweet, shy men in positions like this. I, for one, approach such people apologetically, and always give away the store. In this case, I was acting on the assumption that, because I couldn't fulfill the immigration requirements (permanent residence) of my contract, I would ask the favor of staying on till the end of the semester. I'll go quietly then, suh! The Dean, equally apologetically, asked what if the Immigration Department notified the school, and I guessed it would take some time, we'd already be in semester, and an appeal to let me slide past would make more sense then.

Now in fact, from another perspective, I came to Griffith University in good health but received rather shoddy treatment from the start (no orientation, neither personal, institutional, or otherwise). While working, I took ill, first psoriasis, then full-blown HIV. These are both acknowledged to be stress-triggered conditions. Perhaps my employers (and the state) have some greater responsibility than I have assumed. How have I allowed myself to internalize this guilty attitude which makes me apologize for being ill, and promise to disappear so quietly?

January 17, 1988

Spent yesterday in hospital getting a blood transfusion. No metaphor here: just simple direct vampirism. Read through *Art & Text* "Art Brut" issue, which seemed oddly appropriate to my circumstances. I'm impressed with what amounts to a very formal scholarship displayed by Allen Weiss, but perhaps by many of the authors and, as I think on certain other issues, other writings as well.

Postmodern criticism (if that's what it is) is not raving, signification gone wild. Rather, the complexities of reference and citation revive a nearly medieval scholasticism—a manuscript world. After all, only a few hundred people at most read this (or any such) journal; we write mostly for each other. What's interesting is that this happens at the very moment when the new communications technology celebrates instantaneous access to a global mass audience. But we (provincial academics? scholars? intellectuals?) not only don't have access to this technology to disseminate our work, but the resultant increased price of books, writing materials, and research itself constrains us thoroughly, so we end up circulating our tracts (xeroxed, to be sure) around small, monastic networks alone. Having a journal is a great accomplishment, but our journals are closer to handicraft than mass media. Pressuring Paul to get four color plates in the next issue reminds me that we haven't come so far. The blood took 14 hours to transfuse, but the hospital stay was otherwise without incident.

January 19, 1988

They've just banned an athlete for "topping up"—taking massive blood transfusions before a competition to increase oxygen and energy.

Received a bizarre phone call from this month's AIDS Council student social worker, apologizing because his boss, Peter North, hasn't returned/won't return my call (for three weeks now). I said, "Who put you up to this?" He was very nice and started to have a nervous breakdown on the phone. He promised me a great depth of personal commitment. I said, you're very nice, but far too young for me. It really does not enrich my dying days much to know that I am providing meaningful life experiences for somebody's work-study students at the University of Queensland.

January 20, 1988

Called social worker Alison yesterday to say I was feeling suicidal and crazy: Did any counseling services exist, now that it was clear QuAC was worthless? She gave me the number of a woman, but was a bit vague about who she worked for. Turns out she's the Queensland Health Department and she "already knows everything about my case," and then dropped a few intimate tidbits. Abject paranoia! I've fallen into the trap.

Though she made an appointment, I thought I'd discuss it with Dr. K. when I went in for bloods this A.M. First, he stabbed himself with my needle, then let mine fall from the vein and got a big spray of blood.

Then a call telling Dr. K. that one of the AIDS patients had suicided . . . and what should the police and coroner be told? Not a good morning.

On his advice, I did go for my chat to the Health Department. Nice folks, professional enough to know how to keep me talking. There isn't much they can do except assist me in sinking QuAC, if that's my aim. Dr. K. was intrigued by the politics of all this when he called this arvo.

Stuff it (and the full-time job of being an AIDS victim)! I'm off to Sydney for a week. Only Paul called and said John had been trying to reach me, hadn't left a key, but would be back in Sydney tomorrow night (and so, I don't have flat to myself—may not have a flat at all). If I didn't have leftover work I'd promised to do, I'd have canceled the trip. Chances look good I'll land in the street again. Shit!

January 24, 1988

It's not going badly; I'm not out on the street. Ross picked me up from the airport, took me to *Art & Text* office and then Paul's. John got back from Canberra late afternoon, and I shifted over there.

Not entirely sure what John was up to, why he had to get back to Sydney. . . . Perhaps to give me his key? And then discover he didn't want to go back? In any case, we had a lovely couple of days. Went out to see Ethyl Eichelberger: a high-class New York drag act—much enjoyed, though not as memorable as, say, Michael Clark, the British dancer we went to see last year. Apparently, the Festival of Sydney imports one avant-gay act each year (one Italian, one Greek, etc.) and John and I, by attending two years in succession, now have established a personal tradition about going to these things together. And what's odd is that John, who is in some self-conscious "coming out" process, reckons this may be his only public gay event (we'll try to get to the Mardi Gras parade on time this year). What's awfully odd is that this now is true of me in a sense, too.

After such a public, social gay history, I find it strange to have no direct involvement with the gay world, unless you count dying from AIDS and the guys from QuAC who come in and clean for me. I think that is a mistake, but I'm not sure whose. On the one hand, being sick I'd sure like some more collective involvements, exchanges of information about experiences, alternative therapies, a good dish. . . . But also, I'm desperate to flirt. I even occasionally, but only for the briefest moment, imagine sex with a real live other person. How did I give that up so relatively easily? Obviously, it was tied up with my fieldwork and its commitments. But still, it was easier to quit sex than to give up cruising/flirting. I found it completely depressing this week to walk down Oxford Street looking at all the cuties (and they always look cutest when you can't have them, so they all looked cuter still). I tried stopping in at the Albury off-hours—not to pick anybody up (inconceivable), just to be there, but that even was too, too much. I can't manage my flawed countenance, and I know it's only going to get worse. That was one of the things I found oddly on my generally unburdened mind during this week: Do I start chemotherapy and add another layer of medicalization, routine, and poison cures which further confound my ability to judge sensually my own condition? Or do I let myself degenerate into a deformed and frightening creature? Or is there an alternative? How much brown rice can you eat, anyway?

Got the Powerhouse Museum exhibits done and out of the way, at least my part of it. Not at all happy with the train piece, but I doubt it will look any more ad hoc than anything else. There's a grand stuff-up in that Andrew's painting is the ugliest thing I've ever seen and they're not allowed to insert the monitors into it, as contracted. "That's what white people have been doing to Aborigines for 200 years: cutting apart their Dreamings," Hinton is reported to have said. He should have his tongue cut out, slowly.

January 26, 1988

Australia Day and the Bicentenary refuse to be ignored, at least from the vantage of John's apartment in Kings Cross. I watch the Tall Ships thingo on TV. It seems totally to contradict all the myths Australians assert about themselves. Here is Bob Hawke (reduced over the years to a horrid drag-queen cartoon of himself) sucking up to the royals (the future king and queen of republican Australia!) in a setting—a house on Sydney Harbour—constructed, reeking, of signs of class privilege, as these estates all do. I am reminded that the obsession with standards—"export-quality," "world-class"—is a thinly disguised longing for the more clearly stated hierarchies of the monarchy and British class structures. Occasionally we get to glimpse the lumpen jammed onto the foreshore, mostly under the Harbour Bridge, where one of the limited "free" views of this event are available. They appear to be tanking up at an alarming rate for so early in the day. I am more convinced than ever that Australia's current international appeal is precisely that it is the last place in the world where white people still live so well, their dominance (yea, their natural right to it!) unchallenged. This evokes a nostalgia for the 1950s in America and Britain, before the revolution (which went mostly unrecognized because it turned out to be about race and gender and not especially about economics and class at all, which is where the theorists were looking). Finally, the Fleet arrives, the lead ship proudly bearing a huge Coke logo on its spinnaker. . . .

My skepticism about the Aboriginal anti-demonstration is quickly being overcome by the nearly physical need for collective counter-expression. By noon Hawke has taken to lifting lines from Australian of the Year, minor pop luminary John Farnham, who, you will remember, announced as recently as the New Year's Day tele-launch of the year, with tears in his eyes as always, that because his band contained a Pom, an Aussie and a Yank, it must be multicultural too! Hawke already has this fellow writing immigration policy, I suspect.

I had thought that Aborigines would do best simply and totally ignoring these celebrations. That they decided to converge on Sydney, to demonstrate on this day, seemed to mean agreement to participate, typical of the political naivety the movement usually displays. Fifty years ago, on the Sesquicentennial Australia Day, one had to pay the bus fare and put the Abo's up (albeit, in a makeshift jail). Today, they provide their own fare and swags. A great step forward in self-management. Minister [for Aboriginal Affairs] Gerry Hand was pretty clever supporting these demonstrations, and thereby implying that they too were official Bicentennial events. The only thing remaining was to include them on the printed programs. Still, one cannot deny involvement, and then I've arranged to meet Liz there (who I haven't seen this trip), and I expect I'll find some friends, maybe even Yuendumu folk.

The instructions are a bit vague. "White Supporters" are to meet at Belmore Park and join the march there at 1 P.M. (or 2, or 11—there are contradictory stories, partly because Paul Coe, they say, has declared his own march earlier, perhaps to clear the parade route). And we're to wear black. Now, why whites should wear black isn't entirely clear. Are we to blend in? Or is it a sign of mourning? If so, somebody's got the ethnography wrong again. If there's anything that could be justified as a "mourning color" among most groups, it would be mud/ochre white. . . .

Yesterday's rhetoric, provided by the commercial media anticipating this march, became more and more transparently South African; it revolved around the question, put most badgeringly to "radical" (e.g., half-caste) leaders, "Will this march be violent?", where unequivocal no's are met with sequences of hypotheticals (what if the cops shoot your infant child?). The other tactic was to interview some "real" Abo's from out bush, preferably black as the ace of spades, who seemed confused or otherwise equivocal, or simply offered an original viewpoint about the purpose and politics of the demonstration. This makes implicit, or even explicit, that "real" Aborigines aren't protesting the Bicentenary (only "so-called" Aborigines). Hardly surprising that overseas press correspondents will today call Australians, "Just Nazis with Tans!" It is shocking. I find some black clothes and I'm on my way.

A wonderful, wonderful afternoon for an unreconstructed hippie like myself. Probably 20,000 people, which is enough to form a "sea" of people on Sydney's streets and generate whatever sense of ideological and political *communitas* is intended at moments like this. A mild sense of danger: the police have set up blockades through which we may pass "as individuals but not as a group"—are they totally mad? Why play into the hands of the demonstrators? This march could so easily have been totally co-opted if the state had merely provided some balloons and a marching band! But it wasn't. Apparently, nobody ever lost money overestimating racism here. So everybody played their part and the demonstration, from anybody's point of view, succeeded.

We non-Aboriginals (a curious term of whose legitimacy I am not certain) apparently required stage directions. "Would non-Aboriginal people please clear the footpath so that the Aboriginal people can pass by." This, of course, renewed my critical perversity even as I was having a grand time. Part of my pleasure was the discovery that these 20,000 people included a surprising number of the comparatively few white and black people I'd come to know and care about here. Heading the march was a contingent from Central Australia, including Robin and Harry from Yuendumu, all done up in red ochre. They got wonderfully excited when they saw me, only they couldn't break ranks of course. I figured I'd see them later. And then, I'm looking at this old fella, walking along beside a cross(!) who looks to me like Paddy Jupurrurla, and it *is* Paddy Jupurrurla. Unmindful of our stage directions, I rush up, grasping his hand. His eyesight is failing; he doesn't recognize me with the beard. "Japanangka!" I say, indicating myself, "Yurntumuwardingki!" He goes wide-eyed, and bursts into tears. It's Paddy who had Mary write me the letter when he found out I was sick. And then, "Would non-Aboriginal people . . ." and we were separated.

Okay. Politically, I still agreed. I'd see Old Paddy later. But as it turned out, this spatial divisioning of Aboriginals/non-Aboriginals meant that at the very crowded rally, the segregation remained difficult to break. I never got close to Paddy or the other Yuendumu people again. And then came stage direction number two: "Would all non-Aboriginal people leave the shaded areas so that the Aboriginal people can sit there." Now was revealed the true reason for wearing black on an especially sunny, hot Sydney midsummer mid-afternoon.

Yet the Australian left, or what's left of it, seems to expect, rather welcome, this kind of treatment from Aborigines. If they'd been asked to wear dog shit, they'd probably have complied. That's what's so weird. Do they imagine this public self-mortification compensates for their utter failure to advance any further than a liberal antiracism (antiapartheid rock concerts), and their failure to specify a radical critique of race's place in the development of Australia's—indeed, of capital's—colonial, and neocolonial history, to see that racism and Aboriginal history are central to any theory of history or political action in Australia?

I blame the left, and the Labor Party, more than Aborigines here, who can be forgiven (but not much longer) for seizing whatever advantages are presented. But even while blacks may so claim some privileged position in this debate, it is a tactical tragedy to co-opt it and exclude the left because it damages that left severely, which they will discover, too late, was really the only support for Aboriginal rights in this unaccountably racist country. It seems a poor indulgence to exhaust land rights' limited support by using white supporters as whipping boys. Overseas support really can only do so much.

But maybe it is not merely naive indulgence on the part of the blacks. One curious result is that the Australian left ends up supporting, encouraging, even backing the rise of the bourgeois black new right—people committed to destroying, among other things, these very lefties. The rule seems to be not merely that one never criticizes a black; one never even discusses Aboriginal politics any more. Maybe this is just an overreaction to the abundance of popular racist discourse (not to mention the desire of people like Perkins and Yunupingu to escape criticism). I think it is terribly risky. Does self-determination now require an exemption from public dialogue? I think the problem has gone beyond solution. One fears that meanwhile the concerned left has contracted into the few thousand people in Hyde Park today (I knew so many of them!), there to offer Gary Foley a chance to quite literally push them around "Out of the Shadows, Into the Sunlight" (the title of a particularly offensive Education Department documentary film on Aboriginal bush schools, ca. 1970). The left probably has no choice but to reconstitute itself as an ethnic group, apply for funding, and try to get an hour on SBS-TV.

Never found Liz (we lunched next day); sat with Kevin K. and gossiped about the Institute of Aboriginal Studies, Willmot, etc. Feeling tired. Almost ready to go back to Brisbane. . . . That's a good vacation!

January 27, 1988

Kiwi criminal/old boyfriend Jim called me at John's, sonofabitch! I basically said I didn't want to talk to him, and hung up. I think this very mature of me. Now I don't have to go on reviewing in my head a whole endless text of dialogic moves, countermoves, etc., which would have come to the same thing anyway. I think now, perhaps more than ever, it is important to have regrets, to admit mistakes (don't you just hate that "I wouldn't do anything different" bullshit . . . hell, it's clear I should have been a dyke!) and to cultivate carefully a few feuds—to identify and maintain at least one or two people you will refuse ever to speak to again. Jim made himself such a worthy candidate for this status, why deny it to him? One doesn't meet such assholes every day (article of faith number 347).

January 30, 1988

One might imagine that one will be happy to get back to Brisbane. Then the phone rings, the post arrives. Then the doorbell chimes, then the people upstairs have a party, and the people downstairs try and drown them out with their mega-stereo. You go out to get your washing and it's been nicked off the Hills Hoist (the total collapse of the social contract). You find yourself spending hours calling interstate, overseas, but unwilling to answer when the phone rings. You finally find your employment contract, and discover an ironclad two-week dismissal clause. It's only a matter of time. No wonder you run from the house screaming. No wonder.

February 2, 1988

It's getting more and more difficult to look in the mirror as the KS begins to claim my face beyond the mask of the dreadful but unavoidable beard. I shall not be able to visit the States; I won't get through customs. I won't be able to lecture, as my condition will be too horrible and revolting. I won't be able to walk down the street without attracting attention. What a nasty, nasty disease this is—relentless in its strategies, and always a step ahead of you, winning against any minor attitudinal or medical successes one tries to claim. As the big AIDS conference was taking a very humanist line in Britain, a gay couple with what the press described as "tiny" facial KS lesions, was denied entry at Heathrow airport. I've been invited home for Passover. (Already, sister Jill objects and proposes subversive counterplans that have me flying all over the States. . . . She will have to be educated, but already I suspect we will be unable to construct the illusion of family even for this limited purpose.) I wonder if I can go.

February 4, 1988

Dr. K. came over and discussed my lesions last night. We'll try and do something nontoxic with as many as we can, but the solutions are limited, partly through my continuing poor cell counts. Interesting: a readout of my cell counts over the last six months shows that I was in better shape in September than I thought. Classic KS; probably no opportunistics; best prognosis of the full-blown category. Then, in October–November, something really did happen and my system nearly totally collapsed. It has recovered more apparently than objectively, as my cell counts still don't look particularly good, except where it's vampire blood, not mine, being tested. Oh well.

Lee and I go to dinner and to see what we thought would be *Tenue de soirée* (which I didn't really want to see again, but I did want Lee to see) because we had arranged to see *Caravaggio*, but then it wasn't playing. We were somewhat into the movie (an uncut, explicit fucking scene) when I realized this wasn't a trailer for a coming attraction but the main feature, which, somehow I realized soon after was *Betty Blue*—which I didn't think I'd mind seeing, but hadn't expected. Bugger these repertory art cinemas! Well, I did mind seeing it. Two hours in the sordid lives of the heterosexuals. How difficult they made it all seem. But then, to be manipulated by the characterological involvements and the arbitrary rhetorical narrative moves that lead one to ask such things as, "Why did he kill her?"—as though we had forgotten that she, and he, are only actors pretending in line with their instructions from a director and writer who have made all this up. I really don't want to care about any of this. What makes this French Gothic/Young Wertheresque movie appeal to the university audience (who at U.Q. proved to be into smart-assness, and I was impressed with Griffith's enrollment all over again)? All my little precious preciouses must fear they will uncover some similar flaw deep within that will drive them crazy too, or already has! What rubbish! It was rubbish even in 1966 when I went to university and thought I was mad, too.

February 7, 1988

Need to resist the tendency to lapse into the gray fog of lazy, pointless days: reading pap books (even Gore Vidal) and every weekend newspaper published in Australia.

Was on the phone to John and mentioned I was about to miss seeing *Caravaggio*; he said don't, and it proved the only way to get off the phone. I'd been a bit put off by Lee's report that dreadful Grahame and class traitor Gary were disappointed because it wasn't really gay. Quoting Will Brito, who, when asked if he was gay, replied "Gay? . . . I'm hysterical!", *Caravaggio* is hysterical, at least in the sense that it is absolutely about what being gay is about: maleness, femaleness, competition, status, class art and artifice.

But I do begin to wonder how I feel so free to claim such absolute authority regarding just what is gay. The pluralism of my model itself seems a rationale ("socially, the genius of homosexuality is how it manages to bring so many different people so variously recruited into play on a single gameboard"). But I keep encountering unfamiliar and unclassifiable homosexualities. Indeed, Gary, for example, strikes me as a (ugh!) heterosexual man who happens to fuck boys for whatever reasons. On the other hand, Brisbane seems oversupplied with obvious queens who are married and apparently heterosexual functionally. And then there is John's situation (or Rick's): committed to gay identities but having considerable difficulty finding one. Something more complex than mere pluralism is at work here. But then, I have to admit that even I rarely sustained my preferred democratic/Whitman version of desire.

Spent all night on the phone, mostly the Centre: Philip and Marcia, Peter. All told, I spent three hours today on interstate long-distance. Any day, the three-month bill will arrive. I am prepared for $1,000. Anything more, I'll just die!

February 9, 1988

Perhaps it would be good for our digestion, our health, or our souls if once a month (maybe once a year would be enough) we forgave somebody who in the past we had mentally convicted of unforgivable crimes. If so, then I would be inclined to nominate Paul Simon for the first such dispensation from my "Hall of Hate" after watching the broadcast of his Graceland concert.

We needn't review Simon's crimes; they are heinous and date back over an unimaginably long time, at least to the release of the unspeakable "I Am A Rock," ca. 1966. (He was a rock, too.) But forgiveness implies forgetfulness. The confused politics of his current work aren't any clearer, either. Did Graceland break ranks with an international boycott? At least here in Australia, it was impossible to ascertain the issues, and so the anti-apartheid movement must be faulted equally: if they had an issue, they failed to articulate it despite the enormous publicity Simon was getting. (I had suggested boycotting his concert here, but found out I'd be all alone, again.)

Still, there must be an award for bravery for this pudgy, middle-aged bourgeois Jewish New Yorker for getting up on stage alone, in only black jeans and a white T-shirt (though rather too carefully turned up at the sleeves) and attempting to look cool, even hip, in a sea of Africa's premier black natural rhythmists. He managed it in an appropriately modest, even self-effacing manner, but broke, as things progressed, into a few gestures of play, awkward glee, self-conscious grace.

Australia totally lacks this African input and the resultant cultural dialogue, which is precisely the circumstance of my own growing up in Philadelphia. Allen Ginsberg used to date the shift from Beat to

Hippy as a shift from Black to Amerindian cultural imitation among white youth. But really, the privileged position of blacks always remained in the definition of what was cool, what was sophisticated, in language and performance, at least for my (and adjacent) generations of white Americans. Blacks seemed to have—without even trying—everything we tried for and lacked: cultural certainty, grace under pressure and threat, rich social networks, great dance styles, and big dicks. It's so odd for me to try and reconstruct the experience of growing up in Australia in the 1950s and 1960s (as most of my current friends did) without this model, without this black influence. And now that Australia watches American blacks endlessly on imported sitcoms, what on earth can they be making of these images? How on earth do they relate to Bill Cosby, Nell Carter, J. J., and all the others who now populate their TV world like visitors from another planet?

Doesn't look like I'll be accepting Dad's invitation to Passover at Cape Cod. A scheduling problem at school makes that week perhaps the only really impossible one in the whole year. I had thought, what the hell, my employers should allow me my one chance to get home and see my family before I die. But actually, I now feel more resentful that my family can't seem to work out their own traveling and holiday agendas to accommodate me. So, I guess I'll stay put.

February 11, 1988

I'm 40. Ho hum! It doesn't seem especially consequential from here. I spent the better part of the day answering the phone: Liz, John, Françoise(!), Penny, Dr. K. And went into hospital to get my antibiotic script filled, since I ran a high fever last night.

Dinner with Julie J.-B., up from Sydney for the day on work. Liz had just told her about my condition; I talked far too much, I'm sure, and ordered her the crayfish without even checking the price, knowing she'd pick up the check. Well, at least I only had soup. Sat high above the city, looking down at it, always the best perspective from which to curse Brisbane, which this week I am calling "sleazoid capital of the earth." What's odd is that I got no cards or calls locally, saw no one, talked to no one. When Julie asked if I hadn't expected to hate Brisbane, I said that I've never particularly hated any place, so I didn't expect it, and worse, didn't know how to deal with hating it. To be fair, Lee and Stuart are throwing a party for me tomorrow night. I gather Philip won't make it in till Saturday, though, so he'll miss it.

February 12, 1988

The mystery of Françoise's calls is solved. Sure, we were close, but I find her present attention odd in some way—after all, for two years she never wrote or answered my inquiries. But I got a letter from Pam D. (who's in Canberra now, not Alice Springs), which describes her shock at hearing about my illness, and which occasions this statement of support for me and my work. I get many such remarkable letters now. They're wonderful and they're scary; wonderful in what they say, scary in that they seem to represent some sort of genre/ritual—a little like looking up from your bed and discovering a priest giving final rites.

But guess who told Pam? Françoise, who I gather has now fashioned herself as the Canberra/A.N.U. expert on my condition. I don't mean to be cruel, but I am reminded of my disagreements with Françoise over her fieldwork and publication ethics, and cannot help thinking I am now being subjected to the same insensitivity.

Got letters from Dennis and Calvin in reply to my recent announcement to them. These, Dennis's especially, may be American variants of that genre. Yet this is less obvious, partly because the effort of Dennis's letter is so clear, as though he's holding my face in his hand and forcing my full attention. Slap, slap, slap.

February 15, 1988

A birthday weekend, and some quite lovely things happened. Friday night, Lee and company arrived at the door with a portable instant party and we had a sociable time for a few hours. Met Toby, new tutor in our teaching group, who, it turns out, taught with John in Sydney last semester, and seemed very anxious to be friendly. Good, I could use some friends. Midway into the party, Athol called to tell me that the Institute had voted me a six-month salary. My ticket out of here! There remains some complex bargaining to be done, but still. . . . And the indication of support is breathtaking. No dissension on the Board, according to Athol. Now, I can't honestly believe that certain individuals have suddenly reassessed me and my work and suddenly decided they like/approve/value me. There must be at work some additional consideration that people cannot avoid in situations like this. It becomes a matter of honor, if not karma, to conduct oneself well in the presence of death. How they treat me somehow has implications for their own future.

Philip finally got here from Alice Springs on Saturday. He was coming down with tonsillitis and much of the weekend was spent trying to deal with that, to get a doctor and medications. Still, we had a good rage: by Sunday morning we were calling each other crypto-fascists and screaming our heads off. I can't think of anything I could do that could be more reassuring to Philip, and was glad to see him actually getting quite angry, at which point I backed off. But there's some horrid paranoid logic that infects Alice Springs, and it's very hard for people to pull out of it, or its rigid contradictions. He asked me to take on a language policy project for Imparja Television. I don't think I'll have the time or stamina, and I have to examine the implications of doing so (e.g., can I still do my critical paper with Liz?), but it's so very important I agreed to look at their proposal. I did think it was partly a symbolic offering as well; I'll see how much so.

No phone calls all weekend. Liz is in Hawaii, John wasn't home, and Ross called about *Art & Text* business, but I deferred it till today. I feel irrationally hurt by the failure to launch the monograph, and of the deterioration of my relations with Paul in general.

February 16, 1988

Agro starting up again. This makes me notice it had gotten comparatively quiet for a few weeks, or maybe only days. But the war with the downstairs neighbors began full tilt a few minutes ago when they appeared at my door to complain about me banging on the floor, which was my New York way of complaining about the volume of their music. Why do I have to listen to Rod Stewart, for crissake! But there is simply no way to negotiate these things where people believe they are endowed with certain inalienable rights: to carry guns, to find the perfect match, to play their stereos loud after 11 P.M. . . . I'd move tomorrow, if it weren't the worst time for flat hunting, which is horrible any time, and expensive, and I may be able to get out of here altogether in a few months—which then makes taking another lease impossible, transferring utilities, etc., etc. Stuck again.

Meanwhile, the Institute's miraculous offer of a secondment and salary (which makes escape feasible) may itself go down in a sea of agro. The Dean is already calling me up with all the impossibilities "he hadn't thought of" when Athol and I presented the plan to him. I simply can't believe that they couldn't resolve everything and take good care of me if they were motivated, or simply competent.

Yesterday, I found myself finally unable to jerk off at all—after two days of trying, after nearly a week of not bothering. In the last months, my ejaculate had reduced to a thin, clear, and difficult-to-provoke minimal stream lacking any propellant force at all. Now even that's gone. I suppose, then, that's that. One wonders to what degree this is a physiological nonresponse, and to what degree it's emotional. Getting excited—fixing on an object of desire—is the first hurdle. It is indeed difficult to muster much narcissism, and simply none of my pornography is even minimally credible any more. Even so, it's probably more precise to say that I turn myself off than that I don't turn myself on.

I do not, of course, fully comprehend these mechanisms of desire. I suspect one can't; this, too, melts if you fix long enough on it. I do know that I always require an image—if only a fleeting fantasy—of some other. Even when jerking off I could never (except maybe in adolescence) produce a totally mechanical, self-generated orgasm. As with so much of sexual mystery, I wondered in what way this was or wasn't true of everybody. I recall looking down (or up, in rarer cases which seem, in this instance, quite different) during sex into certain frenzied faces and suspecting, with an equivocal, but alienated chill, that my partner's palpitations were suspiciously out of synch. But I still, in some sense, envy those people who might really be able to claim "it's just friction," which refers to my teenage misreading of Reich. Sexual desire—for me defined by resistance, constraint, exclusion, canalizing—would, when unfettered, become truly an unconscious bodily function. Of course, it was anything but. Anyhow, such hyperbisexuality (even more, sexuality without object) probably is very suspect and may well be associated with pathology. The politics of desire insists that sex must always recognize and then activate difference. Not to mention the economics: the requirement to limit one's cruising to a defined population. Nothing is more dangerous than somebody who cannot differentiate, say, men from women (or, conversely, who can fragment the self to create an internal difference capable of producing a truly autoerotic friction).

In my case, coming to terms with that took a long time. At first (by which I mean "coming out" circa 1972, New York) my motives were various, my desires somewhat diffuse. I was surprised that my sexual relations with women so abruptly halted after I walked into the Gay Activist Alliance firehouse. But it was years before I could actually be said to lust after men, after masculinity, after cock (or ass? . . . how does that compute here? am I confusing phallocentrism again?). Only by 1976, in Austin, Texas, had I come to the point of obsessive lust: expecting sex every day, usually twice a day, and three or four times seemed hardly excessive. Of course, what counted as sex varies; let's say orgasm with different partners. It's not accidental that I achieved this in Austin, not New York, or San Francisco, or even Philadelphia (where, when in residence, I led a more sedate life). It was precisely the absence of a well-defined gay world that encouraged my promiscuity. In big-city fag scenes, I was more critical, more careful, more fearful of being sucked into something impossible to extricate oneself from. I do think Austin was a far more civilized place to be a whore. Local etiquette maintained all sorts of positions for redemption and reclamation, salvation and backsliding, and so I could imagine that I never lost it (control? self? ambition?) completely, irrevocably, as would surely happen in New York, where the competition was, at the same time, more frenzied and demanding, and the definitions (artist/model, agent/star, producer/consumer) so irresistible.

By 1977, of course, my life was a total wreck. I was obsessed wholly with maintaining the balancing act between desire and desirability. I came to regard career—hell, even paying the rent!—as a trade-off against sexual adventurism, and eventually I had to do something to limit my hedonism. In that sense, it sounds rather like what I had done with LSD (or what LSD did to me) in the previous decade. Indeed, in both cases, there was an attempt to make a theology and a politics out of the habit—which should not be dismissed or repudiated even here. My paltry solutions included attempts to make steady boyfriends more desirable . . . in principle, but in reality the same disaster as ever. Lord, am I lucky that I had no taste for heroin or physiologically addictive drugs! I recall invoking a set of rules which insisted that I view other things as more important, at any given moment, than getting laid. For example, if there was anything at all to do on a given night rather than go to the gay bars, I was committed to do it. Just imagine how much sex there was in those 1970s that you had to make rules to distract yourself in order to get anything done: the statistics are just staggering! Surely, such opportunities arise only rarely in human history—and are bound to be abrogated by epidemic disease.

I do tend to see my current disease as a kind of cosmic personal reducing plan, where one by one certain functions disappear. But unlike LSD, which I argued rendered inoperable only undesirable functions (like rational thought, the ability to complete a sentence), I see no necessity in the particular direction of AIDS's progress. To the contrary, the only available strategy is reduced to trying to exercise preferences as to the order of loss involved. I prefer to jettison the sex, for example, in preference to the memory, indeed any other mental functions. There may be some economy of energy to consider as well. I assume thinking burns up less calories.

I have always rejected the idea that gay promiscuity stems from some inherent biological drive of the male (finally released to a world of unlimited opportunity). Instead, promiscuity acknowledges the fragility of the gay identity, the constant necessity to reassert homosexuality precisely because it is not a persona, a practice, a sociability learned and acquired in infancy (as heterosexual forms are thought to be), rewarded and reinforced in familial and all other institutional contexts throughout childhood and youth. Homosexual forms—transactable gay identities, negotiable desires, how to be gay—probably are learned no earlier than adolescence, and often much later (although the psychological aetiology and even the "choice"—in whatever sense it is one—to be gay may reach back further still). Gayness remains emergent in social action, and may never quite become internalized, so that each night we seek to rediscover that identity by performing those rights of hyperexchange based on rituals of endless, byzantine moves whose purpose is definitional at least as much as it is the trading-off of sperm (an objective which in homosexuality itself is largely symbolic in its transformation of natural to cultural purposes).

If I don't now do any of these things, if I can't even jerk off, to what extent can I be said to be gay? The question arose first for me when I moved out to the Central Australian Desert. One could also count earlier visits with my parents on Cape Cod where for days, even weeks, all contact with the gay world was severed by distance and immobility. I would come out of those visits so ultrasexed I remember thinking I could fuck a sheep in the New York subway. Why a sheep, why the subway, remains a mystery to me, probably an indication of how warped the imagination can become on these parental visits. At Yuendumu, something else happened, over time. In the beginning, I would arrange to get down to Sydney every few months for a weekend, and then, look out daddies! I knew what cowboys felt like when they got into Dodge after months on the range. I barely had time to talk. Curiously, during three years of this, I barely met anybody (except Martin), never was invited home, went to any parties, etc., etc. The fault was mine; I didn't have time to date. When back in the bush, I carefully nurtured a small gay video collection (safer than magazines), and used to cherish the rare occasions of privacy that provided an opportunity to jerk off to them (privacy soon becomes the most cherished and rare commodity for the modern Westerner living in most tribal societies). I developed quite elaborate relationships with my video images. But over time, even this novelty wore off. Something curious happened also to my appearance; I stopped posing in mirrors or considering my cosmetology. I felt quite liberated in some sense, acknowledged that what mirrors were available was the community itself, and yet I was limited in my ability to read those mirrors. By the end of the fieldwork, my gay identity was problematized and backgrounded in ways I never could have imagined, let alone tolerated, five years before. It has made the transition to enforced celibacy easier. But if psychologists are right about the centrality and fixation of identity for the human self, what terrible psychic violence something like AIDS must wreak on most gays—and has perhaps done to me, although my analysis seems to offer a particular exemption for my case on this count, if only to rationalize and distance myself from the sad fact that I expect never again to engage in those caresses of the body which sustained and defined me for most of my adult life.

Had my first radium treatment today. Another few hours of medical bizarrerie. In this case, the therapy room had the same bucolic wall mural I had used to kitsch up my last flat. Fortunately, they asked me to close my eyes during treatment.

February 19, 1988

Wednesday afternoon. Margaret Reilly called from the Warlpiri Media Association [WMA] to say that they were unhappy with the photo to be used on the cover of *Art & Text*. I was appalled; it should already have gone to press! I told M. there was probably little that could be done, but I'd call the publisher. Ross was his usual bemused/amused competent self. The plate had been struck and should be printed Friday. Maybe it could be replaced before then. And it could be defaced, selectively. We had fun with substitutions. Paul wanted a label, "This penis has been censored by request of the Yuendumu Community Council." I submitted the less insulting (but more trite), "Ceci n'est pas un pénis."

I called Margaret back to ask if it was the whole thing or merely the phallic graffiti that bothered them. She'd have a meeting and ask them, and get back to me on the morrow. Thursday she called back in the afternoon to say they had decided they didn't want the graffiti published at all. I had earlier explained that I asked people's indulgence in this, as the penalties to me of withdrawing the picture at this point would prove totally out of proportion to the act; I'd be in big trouble, my publisher, the Institute, my salary, etc., etc. But I doubt Margaret understood, let alone represented my position. Even more, the article accompanying the picture asserts as analytic text exactly the same points the picture makes. They'd had the text for months. Didn't anyone read it? Obviously, they don't want that published either, even if they don't know it. I told Margaret, "Okay, would you let people know that I want nothing more to do with the WMA." Margaret started to jack up, saying I had no right and I countered that it was the only right left to me.

Many things are going on here. First, I have to acknowledge that I provoke these crises, very much on purpose. By pushing into especially difficult and contradictory areas of modern Warlpiri life, I assure these confrontations. And I imagine that pursuing these has some pedagogic value for Yapa [Warlpiri people], as much as for me. In this case, the WMA is making an appeal for power by analogy to media restrictions and controls based on traditional laws governing secrecy and death (which we articulated during my work there). But now, I think these are being applied to a wholly secular question of community PR/self-image (Christian Tidy Town). Undoubtedly, by encouraging media controls, I helped set up the very environment in which this transference could occur. At the same time, I think this strategy is dangerous and self-defeating (beyond just the offense to free speech—which I may find distasteful, but also maybe so what!). It seems especially bad tactics to exercise these controls only on people who offer themselves up for consultation, because they continue to have no power over the majority of outsiders who never submit a thing for comment or vetting. In fact, I enjoy these fights; they keep me feeling alive. But somehow this one seemed more upsetting, and provoked my extreme response and withdrawal (although I intend that as a move in a game which I mean to keep open, although I may find the game has finished and nobody else thinks we're still negotiating).

What I think bothers me so much is that I am being denied a position in the debate, an existence in the community, an identity in the political sphere of Yuendumu which I had reason to think had been earned, acknowledged. This is why I take it totally personally, as an act of betrayal (as, I suspect, a Warlpiri man would also). I felt dismissed. My appeal to my small area of expertise (which is precisely media circulation and art marketing) is denied, and the additional claim that this is very important to me is ignored. Finally, the extreme efforts I've gone to to pull them out of the poo on some recent projects is not acknowledged and no reciprocity is extended.

I take it personally because this is my reading of how these things are in fact understood in Warlpiri. But, examined more closely, I think I have a number of responsibilities here. It is a bad, and dangerous, mistake to seek to censor for mere rhetorical and public relations purposes. In the case of art in particular, exclusion from criticism will mean exclusion from the "serious-consideration market," and reversion to tourist kitsch markets. My obligations as expert, as adviser, as participant in Warlpiri media seem to require that I maintain my position here, even at considerable risk, so that these issues become clear for the community, and to resist the thuggery that I detect in Margaret and certain Japangardi.

Obviously, this has further inflated my phone bill. I've spoken for 30 minutes or more with Penny (strictly speaking, it's her photograph), with Peter Toyne, with von S. (twice), Mary L., Ross, etc. Everything else stops abruptly as these matters demand full attention.

I'm still not certain what to do. If the photo was mine, I'd be very tempted just to bully it through. Again, I believe it is dangerous if WMA comes to believe it can claim powers of control above those that either

Aboriginal or common law recognizes. And so, I must be the provocateur. But the picture isn't mine and although Penny was going to release it to me, I advised her against it. This is precisely the sort of issue the Institute isn't equipped to handle and Penny can't afford to confront. I expect I'll ask Ross if he can substitute one of my slides, not notably different in content, merely mine. This may, or may not, look like a compromise more than I intend. We'll see. As it will be some time before the thing actually comes out, any immediate debacle might defuse by then. But I think I'll make it clear that I see no requirement to vet my photo in this case, even if that's provocative.

I will need to explain to Paul and Ross, at least, that this is just what I do for a living, and there really isn't anything extraordinary about it.

February 21, 1988

6:30 A.M. I was just awakened by a banging on the door. I lay in bed and listened to it, incredulous since nobody I know would visit at this hour. When I arose and answered it, it turned out to be one of Brisbane's finest with a warrant for my arrest, demanding $78.25 or he'd haul me off to jail. He wouldn't tell me at first what I was being fined for (failure to wear a seat belt?); I was just to pay the money. It did have a date, sometime in April last year. Since the social worker, Alison, arranged to clear all my fines in November, something was obviously wrong here. I was not nice. I did have $80 in hand, but he didn't have change, and told me to stop by the station later. None of this fits with any notion of due process in my book. I said, you know, there are countries where policemen show up at the door at these odd hours demanding money and threatening people without telling them what for; I didn't think this was one of those countries. As ever, his final, devastating comeback was, "Why don't you go back where you came from!" I think I shall hold a competition to develop alternate comebacks for that remark. "Practicing for the [Brisbane] Expo?" is wearing a bit thin.

February 28, 1988

Another week in Sydney. In a way, it's now more like attending to a parallel life than visiting some other place. Nothing monumental happens; I don't strain myself. Merely, I lead a busy, social, engaged life, as opposed to Brisbane. It makes returning unpleasant, excepting the opportunity to crawl into my own bed, my cotton sheets, and reclaim my local territory (it seems the downstairs rockers have fled, making this a somewhat more bearable prospect).

Paul agreed to go with a substitute cover, one of my slides, for the magazine, and then required me to write a 100-word statement for the back cover. I am to feel complimented; only Baudrillard, I think, has had a back cover on *Art & Text* before. But I feel conned. How can I possibly compress the issues to 100 words? Why not just put a picture of me on a rifle target and write under it, "Enemy of the Indigenous Peoples"? But Ross and I worked out a text, sandwiched in between some good quotes from New York subway graffiti artists, which will have to do.

I actually met new people on this trip, something I am so armored against in Brisbane. I simply decided that if my appearance bothered others, it should remain their problem. (Would it really be easier if people asked me point blank, and I could answer, "Cancer . . . ARC"?) Wednesday night was celebrity night, dinner at the Oxleys' on Darling Point for Paul Taylor. The other half continues to live quite well, thank you. Priceless Lichtensteins in the toilet, the first really classy salad I've had in Australia, and jokes about stealing the houseboy. It set up a discussion between me and John about the politics of privilege. (Question: Why is Paul Taylor Paul Taylor and I'm not? Answer: He comes from money in the first place.) In fact, I suspect one contradiction at the heart of my family was that my mother convinced us we too came from money, but Daddy never gave us much. I wonder how that feeds my sister's resentment, or was responsible for giving me airs? Paul T. proved to be charming; I wonder if he realizes what a problem he poses for all of us, especially Foss, who must have great difficulty handling his feelings here? Foss responds by overcompensating, I suspect, being overly gracious, and finally risking acting a grotesque cartoon of the pimp. We are, after all, nasty street queens and shall never achieve that "respectability"; consequently, we must be honest, or at least believe ourselves to be—which queers any chances of a Darling Point of our own. And so it's no good complaining, is it?

I enjoyed meeting Jim Waites rather more. He seems quite mad, and charming, and his Kings Cross household is comfortably incoherent. He makes a good salad, too, and his sister is sharp as a tack—encouraging for one so young. Was he really Patrick White's lover? Before or after he fell off the cliff and lost his mind? It results in a very appealing asymmetry of thought and countenance. Martyn, the book reviewer, was likewise engaging, and I'm astonished how quickly my condition and disabilities are forgotten in these lovely chatty encounters. Only, I am quite nervous about getting the [Sydney Gay & Lesbian] Mardi Gras piece written for Jim. It makes it worse, not better, that I think he'd be very nice about my failure if it came to that.

Coffee with old boyfriend Martin went on for hours. He looks good, and I'm not sure that it is any more than my own projection which detects an anger and panic under his cheerful surface. We swapped symptoms and solutions, something I really do miss being able to do, but I doubt Martin was cheered by this. He is far more involved in support and discussion groups in Melbourne. I suspect I depressed him, and we didn't manage to get together again, as both of us were busy.

Mardi Gras was remarkable. Unfortunately, I missed most of the events I was supposed to review/attend leading up to it. Couldn't get away from the dinner party in time, misread the schedule, etc. Only got to the Vito Russo talk, walking out in fury after the first half. How can anybody live in New York and be so dumb about the problematics and politics of representation? Why is he Vito Russo and I'm not? Can't Sydney gay life extricate itself from U.S. cultural domination/definition? Apparently not; can anybody? Was gayness really invented only once, in New York circa 1969, so everything else is diffused from there?

I had by Friday intended a critical piece totally slamming these alien sources and the current ethnic bureaucratization of Mardi Gras. But then there was the event, and it was overwhelming. A huge, elaborate parade: it takes a fairy to make it nice. Nobody else could (or, more to the point, would) mount such a spectacle, despite the New South Wales government's penchant for potlatches. It begins to rival the opening celebration of the Olympics. The conspicuous involvement of many women, blacks, and ethnics can't really be criticized. This was probably the only ideologically correct public display in the whole political muddle of Bicentennial Sydney. But it was the sea of partygoers who followed the parade to the Showground that was the real event—tens of thousands of people flowing down the streets of Sydney for hours, appropriating all spaces between the Cross and the Showground. Astonishing, and unarguably political, though it's impossible to venture a reading of what those politics might be or mean. The world really perched on the edge for a few hours, and could at any moment have collapsed into a black hole in the ground and disappear. As close to the "Day of the Locust" as I expect to see! Consequently, I'm sorry I didn't go to the Showground. But then, this sorrow goes deeper than that; I really didn't have the energy. The crippled boy who couldn't follow the piper. I'm sorry I couldn't go to the ball. I'm sorry I turned into a pumpkin so soon. I'm sorry I don't have a boyfriend, can't even cruise, etc., etc. I'm not sure these sorrows are as unproductive as they seem, though. But without John's tender care through all this I would have very little courage at all.

February 29, 1988

First day of classes [at Griffith University]. Where do these bright-eyed-and-bushy-tailed's come from? I am so deeply cynical about this system of education, its arbitrariness and ideo-illogic. Yet the kids keep coming, and offer some unexpected justification for this employment.

March 2, 1988

Peter called from Yuendumu (at last!) to sort through the graffiti business. It started to get very painful; perhaps this was the first time we'd found ourselves adamant on opposite sides of a morally defined issue. Maintaining opposed positions seemed unbearable, considering how highly we regard each other, how we have cared for each other, and, I suspect, what each other's support has meant in rather profound ways over the years. So, holding my breath, I proposed the sort of politically motivated compromise which I do so very badly, and which always blows up in my face. All right, Peter, I've made it perfectly clear that if the first photo were mine I would have gone ahead and published it. But it wasn't. So you are free to interpret that substitution as a compromise with the community, and we can get on with other business for which we obviously need mutual support. Lee assured me when I told him about it that this was a very astute, mature, political move on my part.

Also spent an hour on the phone with Debbie R., about Fred Myers's response to my critique in *Canberra Anthropology*. She still hasn't had the moxie to read it! I assure her that it was all about me and that she escaped very lightly, though it's interesting to speculate on Fred's motives, since I thought she and I said essentially the same thing. Anyway, I am coming to the conclusion that my wounds from this episode may prove fairly superficial. Oddly, my outstanding worry is to figure out if Fred, in objecting to the title ("If 'All Anthropologists Are Liars . . .' "), understood I was including myself, and adding a final, necessary layer of irony, or whether he excludes me from that class and so operates from a very different reading.

March 7, 1988

My hemoglobin level is shocking; I know this even before the tests are back. For at least the last week I've had to drag myself to and fro. The world is suddenly tilted uphill, and every step positively exhausts me. I have even had to drag myself to the study to write this. But it's not entirely unpleasant. Rather, it's most curious to watch everything slow down, to become oddly dissociated from events, or their pace. Knowing that a few units of blood will correct this, will pump me back up to a more normal rhythm, I somewhat savor the current effect. There are problems: I gave my [Aboriginal] Art paper at U.Q. Friday, and nearly passed out, had to sit down midway through. The two or three people in the (rather big) audience who may have known of my condition must have thought, "How brave!" I doubt the rest would have noticed anything. But as I began to feel sweaty and weak and thought I might keel over then and there, I resisted once again: "Not here, not now. . . . I didn't even want to give this lecture today. Who are these people anyway?"

Ross is up for the weekend for the [Bicentennial] "City as a Work of Art" project, which, despite my shocking lack of energy, livens up the time. It causes me to do two things I normally never would: to go downtown to the Queen Street Mall on Saturday morning, and to go there on Saturday night. It was shamefully dull, by the way. Susan was up also, and we're arranging my monograph launch as part of a Super-8 Film Group event at the Chauvel Cinema next month in Sydney. Good. Only the *Times on Sunday* carried a big piece on Francis and BRACS [Broadcasting to Remote Area Communities Services] and I'd have liked to be able to tie into this rare publicity.

March 8, 1988

A lackey from the Immigration Department called today to invite me in for an interview. They wanted to determine if I qualified for a visitor's (tourist) visa. "A tourist visa?" I said. "Does this mean, for example, I lose my job?" That's so. I asked if they'd had correspondence with Canberra on the matter; indeed they had. These are not at all the terms discussed with Canberra! I asked for some time to sort the matter out, as this had caught me totally unawares. They said, "Let's not draw this out as we did in the original application." An outrageous remark, considering that had they moved efficiently on my case a year ago, none of this would have happened. Something has gone terribly wrong, and the jig may well be up. I got on to Liz, the Gay Immigration Task Force, the Institute, and everyone else I could think of. I have to call them Friday for my next set of instructions. Fortunately, I go in for my transfusion Thursday, and maybe I'll be in better shape to handle this. As it is, I could barely drag myself to my classes today.

But I did drag myself to hear A—— M—— declaim tonight at the Institute of Modern Art [IMA] on the role of the critic, and probably shouldn't have bothered. His performance was shocking—ocker, pandering to what he must have imagined the Brisbane audience to want (and he may not have been wrong, but that is precisely not the role of the critic). He was gratuitous, imprecise, and his adroit handling of the discourses and terms of contemporary criticism in service of some shockingly dumb ideas and superficial thinking raises grave doubts about his other work, which I had always liked, even admired.

Had coffee afterwards with Nick Z., who I hadn't chatted to since his return from his world tour, and who was even more annoyed than I at A——'s performance. He dismissed M—— as a species of pop-culture used car salesman. I find I often agree with Nick's critical tastes while finding his reasons obscure, and feel uncomfortable agreeing too readily with him, as I'm never sure what other theoretical baggage I might be buying into. Still, he has always seemed a convivial ally. The conversation shifted to my filling him in on my situation (of which he seemed wholly uninformed—interesting to see how the school's information networks hold in some directions, not others). He seemed to think the school could be counted on for a more explicit form of support; that indeed, if I approached the Minister, or anybody, for that matter, without some statement from my current employer, it would look odd. I agreed, but thought from the very beginning the situation was foregone (and forlorn). Hence, my appeal to the Institute. I'm willing to be wrong. Certainly, it would make me feel better, even if it's too late to accomplish anything.

Obviously, most activities, projects, etc., now cease while I try to sort this out. Such cruel and unusual punishment!

March 13, 1988

As expected, the weekend was mostly spent trying to straighten out this visa business. I'm gratified how quickly and unequivocally everyone I talked to got furious and pledged their help. Letters should start pouring in on Monday (even Yuendumu has a fax now!). I should think the matter will be resolved in my favor. If not, the Department and the Minister will have been given notice that I won't be leaving quietly. But the effect of all this is so depressing. Thinking about going back to the States only emphasizes how inconceivable that is, but also how terribly vulnerable I am. This inevitably leads to pointless reflections on life-and-the-choices-I-made.

Saturday. Drove myself out to Bribie Island to the Rigsbys' for dinner with them and Nancy W. I needed to get Nancy to go to Coombs to go to the Minister on my behalf (I will not take up diary space with the shameful details of the politics and strategies which engross me in trying to respond to the immigration people and which have consumed my time as well). I don't know that I have great personal or professional respect for any of these particular people. And yet, I had such a pleasant, civilized time. Coincidentally, we were all Yanks, and the conversation did occasionally slip into swapping pop culture readings of these amazing Aussies. But even more comfortable was talking about teaching, about anthropology, insider gossip, E—— W—— (which led to the final subject of the evening: lying, and what liars tell themselves they're doing). This comes much closer to what I came into this profession for, and never get to do in Brisbane. (I really am developing the most hideous attitude about Griffith. I'd better be careful.) Anyway, a good time was had. . . .

March 15, 1988

Paul Keating on TV tonight looked just like Mike Gore, only thinner. For that matter, Mick Young looked like a young Bjelke-Petersen. Wonder what's going on in the Labor Party.

I feel surprisingly unharried by the immigration thing. Everybody, including Griffith, is behaving very, very well indeed. If I actually get through this, I could have six months to coast. It would be the first such period in at least two years totally fixated on an image of Sydney Harbour through the great horizonal swoop of a balcony railing.

Letters from Nashie, Jane, a Françoise paper via Mary, letter from Jill, and a wonderful, amazing letter from John von S. (one of two, actually) responding to the *Canberra Anthropology* thing with Myers. As well as I think I muddled through that exchange, I still think the verdict goes against me, the product of a particularly recalcitrant insecurity of the "what do I know, anyway?" variety against Fred's authoritarian certainties (and more extensive data?). Completed the Chatwin piece [on *Songlines*] and got it off to various people, including Les for publication. Working on Mardi Gras piece, which is a drag because I don't feel I've got much to say, and that's not the advantage I'd hoped. The only other major piece looming is the ANZAAS paper, and that can't be anything less than a major undertaking.

March 17, 1988

Finished the Mardi Gras piece for *New Theatre Australia*, at last. Frightening to consider how much prose I can turn out when I have nothing to say. Still, it's not a bad occasional piece. What struck me as odd, however, is that I wrote completely from the position of an Australian, to the degree that might quite rightly invite criticism for deception. And yet, sitting in the bath just now, I fantasized a reply (for ABC-Radio, as I imagined it):

"As is true of so many here, I was not born in Australia; one has little choice in these matters. But it appears I will die here. My first teachers of Australianism, the old Warlpiri men of Yuendumu, believe that fact gives me certain rights here, which I am entitled to invoke."

Called Jill for her birthday this morning. I find it so surprisingly easy to chat to her, I'm glad to say (ignoring that it costs $2 per minute). The question of "coming home" arises, of course, and I'm so indefinite. I claim it depends on work being available and offered, which probably refers to an impossible condition. But then, what do I think of all that? If I weren't ill, I do think I'd be plotting a return in a couple of years, with some publications and a reputation under my belt, mostly because I expect cultural cringe will ultimately defeat all of us here. But frankly, when I think of the States, I only fantasize watching TV and eating regional specialty food. Hardly a basis for national identity.

* * *

[*The article Eric wrote for* New Theatre Australia *appeared in May 1988, titled "Carnivale in Oxford St." It is inserted here—in slightly modified form—as it clearly belongs with the diary entries of the previous two days.*]

The first contingent roaring out of the dark and onto Oxford Street was the motorcycle cops. Not the Cocteau or even the Genet version; these cops were bearers of light, beaming their mega-headlamps before them, blinding the crowd with a stage technique Grace Jones had perfected in her 1978 cabaret tour. As the irises of more than 100,000 spectators readjusted (estimates vary wildly—it seemed the whole city was out), there was a burst of glitz, a shatter of disco sound, then an improbable assortment of people throwing condoms to begin Sydney's tenth annual Gay Mardi Gras.

What followed, for a full hour and a half, and on into the wee hours of the dawn, beggars description. It was so vast, so diverse, so, so ultra, even compared to previous years. In a number of ways, Gay Mardi Gras came of age in 1988 as a fully civic festival in the grand tradition. No longer just a gay parade, it has become a theatrical event gay people perform as an offering to the city at large.

Oxford Street became a canyon, a sort of valley of flesh as spectators lined not only the walkways, but the awnings, the roofs and windows—like flies to every available surface from the Art Gallery, via Oxford and Flinders, and down to the Showground. Lighting borrowed from club ceilings, smoke and confetti machines, huge amps and speakers, even male strippers, were all hauled out of the first-floor windows and used to spectacular effect up and down the street. Not even San Francisco, New York, or Paris can boast this much glitz per square inch for any single event.

Sydney's Gay Mardi Gras had its humble and political beginnings as a small, radical confrontation celebrating the gay Stonewall riots in New York's Greenwich Village (ca. 1969). The move from the date of that June anniversary, internationally celebrated as Gay Pride Week, to February and the antipodean summer (permitting much more revealing and risqué costumes) was hotly debated in Sydney's den of gay politics in the 1970s. Indeed, the matter still is: Does the Gay Mardi Gras retain any political content? I think it may be possible to read in this year's dramatic events unexpected forms of public politics, and so contradict a general belief that, post-Thatcher, post-Reagan, post-AIDS, gay radicalism is moribund. This interpretation depends upon seeing Mardi Gras for what it has become, an amazing piece of street theater, and by considering the sources of that theater tradition in great pre-Lenten Carnivals of the Middle Ages.

The label Mardi Gras refers to Shrove Tuesday, the day in the Christian ceremonial calendar before Lent begins on Ash Wednesday, ushering in its month of solemnity, sanctity, and deprivation. Drawing upon pagan precedents (the great bear god who emerges annually from hibernation to signal the rebirth from winter with a huge fart), medieval Christians came to reckon the period from Candlemas (February 2), or St. Blaise Day (February 3), or even earlier, the feast of the Epiphany (January 6), as the beginning of a licentious ritual schedule.

If Lent required rigid privation, the Carnival period came to mean the opposite: a chance to indulge to excess, to sin publicly, to turn Christian morality (and symbols and rituals) on its ear. A series of street carnivals, athletic contests, mock royal courts, processions, parodies and satires built up to the ultimate moment of abandon, Shrove Tuesday—Mardi Gras—when the whole world turned upside down.

All this was not as harmless or merely symbolic as it might seem. Political historians have become interested in tracing peasant and tax revolts to these events, and even find antecedents of the French Revolution in rural Carnivales. Le Roy Ladurie recounts in *Carnival in Romans* (1979) that, "Each February (Romans) was the scene of a colorful and animated Mardi Gras Carnival. In 1580 the winter festivals were even livelier than usual; they degenerated into a bloody ambush where the notables killed or imprisoned the leaders of the craftsman party. This blend of public celebration and violence burst like a skyrocket over France." Cultural theorists and students of theater have also recently paid increasing attention to these episodes. What interests them about Carnivale is how these rituals actually dramatize, in a mirrored way, the very structures of the society which they play on.

Folklorists are additionally interested in the communal quality of Carnivale. There is no stage, there is no audience; it is a complete, participatory ritual, of the sort either associated with exotic primitives or the avant-garde theories of Brecht and Artaud. Why does Carnivale persist into the age of TV and mass media? How does it encourage *communitas* in an age of isolated, alienated individualism?

A whole set of such questions could be applied to the events of February 27. That doesn't mean that the drag queens in *haute splendeur* (and 20 kilos of lurex glitter) all had advanced academic degrees in social theory—perhaps only a half dozen did. Or that the organizers of the parade figured out a complicated political agenda and inflicted it on an unwitting public. But, of all social identities, homosexuality is most remarkably connected to performance.

The reasons for this are various and reach back into history. A history of oppression, where people had to hide, to mask themselves in daily life, but also a more positive history of association with the sources and institutions of theater itself. The traditions of transvestite drama go back past Dame Edna, past Shakespeare even, into Noh drama, Balinese dance, tribal ritual. Strictly speaking, these forms involve inversions of gender that may not have so much to do with the kinds of identities and relationships preferred by modern gay women and men. But these inversions undoubtedly created a space in which homosexualities could operate in the past, and which gay men, and women, now claim as a proud heritage.

In many repressive societies, Carnivale was the only opportunity for public cross-gender expression. In the early nineteenth century, American gay men from all over that country followed transvestites to the annual New Year's "Mumming," Philadelphia's local version of Carnivale. Tennessee Williams and others describe a well-known history of gays in New Orleans for the Mardi Gras there. And Rio is notorious in this respect.

Yet none of these are specifically gay events: rather, they are events that permit, include, allow, even celebrate cross-gender displays, but as one among a number of forms. Religious, totemic, and pagan iconography are equally evident, and likewise inverted. Of all Carnivales, perhaps only Sydney's Mardi Gras is exclusively about gender and homosexuality. But, as this year proved, it's also about much more than that.

Overseas visitors report being appalled that Sydney could be so gauche as to celebrate its Shrove Tuesday on a Saturday night. This alone, these purists claim, disqualifies the Gay Mardi Gras from serious cultural consideration. They do not understand that Australia is a staunchly civic state, so that this too may be a valid Australian cultural statement. Seasons begin here not on the celestial calendar of solstices and equinoxes, for instance, but on the first day of the appropriate month. Long weekends supersede any religious calendar.

In fact, the last week in February does signal an important moment in the Australian annual cycle. It is as long as one can draw out the summer "silly" (holiday) season—those very last moments before you simply must return to work (the national equivalent of Lenten privation). Foreigners, those sad creatures entitled to only one or two weeks annual leave, cannot possibly understand this, or the mood that governs the antipodes in late Feburary. A Saturday night Mardi Gras is entirely appropriate and does support a cultural analysis.

The sequence and variety of floats that passed down Oxford Street offer possible clues to a "reading" of Mardi Gras. A listing provides some idea of the diversity here: Gay Immigration Task Force; Pollies Social Club; Sydney Theatre Company; Waratah Deaf Association; New Tradition Dancers (an Asian company); Alice Springs Gay Group ("Hot as Hell"); a group of "Dykes on Bikes" (who were in fact unlabeled, but the name sticks anyway); various AIDS support groups, clinics and collectives; a local bathhouse; a gym; Gays in Aviation; Cronulla Gay Group, and so on.

There were in excess of sixty groups represented, and some acknowledgment is due here of the sheer elaborateness of many floats. Groups had obviously worked months on their costumes and exhibits. And it showed, as was intended; this is no occasion for subtlety. My personal favorite was the huge double-sided living Picasso painting: an ambulatory *Demoiselles d'Avignon* on one side, and an animated *Guernica* on the other! But some of the neoclassical stage sets, imitation boats and airplanes, and heavily glitzed-out disco pub floats were okay too. Gay folk pride themselves on their ability to make things "nice." It seems almost pedantic to make the connection to the medieval craftsman guilds, and yet the comparison isn't forced. There are some very ancient sources here as well.

Recent years saw Mardi Gras dominated by AIDS agencies, AIDS support groups, and PWAS (Persons With AIDS). This reflected the community's concern, even obsession, with its health crisis—fairly and responsibly enough, even if it didn't make for the best and most fun parade. In fact, the attention to AIDS worked both ways. Fred Nile used it to try and stop the parade.

The organizers won that round, and won big by arguing convincingly that the Mardi Gras provides the best available opportunity for desperately needed public information and education.

To some extent, the Australian gay movement (or at least its most articulate personnel) had already been appropriated into the AIDS bureaucracy by this time, and was beginning to feel both the strengths and constraints of its new quasi-official status. It's now several years later; AIDS hasn't gone away by any means, but it no longer dominates the gay scene, its funding, institutions, employment or its discourse. A sort of post-crisis mentality has become possible, expressed, joyfully, in this year's Mardi Gras.

In fact, this may well have been the year of the "multicultural." The participation of Asians, Islanders, and other communities not usually as public, was remarkably visible. The appearance of an Aboriginal float and its position of honor at the head of the line was new. Their parody of James Cook and the First Fleet may well have been the only "politically correct" public event of the Bicentennial year.

Is the gay community jockeying for a position in the new Australian ethnic panoply? Indeed, is it seeking to become a "community" (an issue of definition currently being hotly debated by gay activists and sociologists) by analogy to the national and cultural enclaves we usually mean when we use that term? Are we all "wogs" now? Is that what we saw in this parade (and what made it so successful at the same time)? Certainly this would mean a break with the more elitist, British and royalist styles that have persisted in Sydney's gay world.

Maybe we are merely seeing an opening up or a diversification of gay style. Or are we finally recognizing that this was always there, and that the narrowly defined Oxford Street clone was always a misrepresentation of the more diverse varieties of homosexualities? The parade's one classic clonelike group, a leather contingent—masters and slaves pulling a three-and-a-half-meter-high papier-mâché "macho man" down the street—certainly looked oddly archaic.

Had there been only the "official" parade, these questions of pop sociology might have seemed deceptively easy to answer. But that parade was only a prelude to an even more spectacular parade which invoked the deeper sources and darker power of Carnivale. As the sequins and feathers and stray bits of tulle floated down onto Flinders Street and swirled into the Showground, they signaled the start, not the end, of an even more radical procession.

For fully an hour and a half, tens upon tens of thousands of people streamed into the streets in the first parade's wake; some were headed to the party at the Showground (indeed, one had little choice of direction in this flow of humanity). But some seemed more involved just with taking over the streets. For two hours after the parade passed, something really approaching Carnivale happened, until the police attempted to regain control and the council workers tried to reclaim Oxford Street for the more sensible elements of Sydney.

Authentic Carnivale, like other ritual theater, does not separate spectator from event, audience from actor, across the boundary of the proscenium arch. This is one of the sources of the power of ritual theater. Everyone is drawn in; safe, defensible lines are breached. This defines a site of danger, excitement, and political potential like no stage show can.

This is what "Act 1" of the Gay Mardi Gras parade lacked. There, the boundaries were drawn: street/walkway; revelers/audience; us/them. Probably these boundaries are necessary to permit Mr. and Mrs. Suburbia to be spectators at a gay event comfortably. But with the last float, the line collapsed, and for a remarkably protracted moment, all boundaries, social as well as spatial, were up for grabs.

For a gay festival, this moment is especially telling, and challenging, because the line between gay and straight is itself so vague. Members of ethnic and other special communities mostly are recruited at birth, and remain identified and identifiable throughout life. The line between "us" and "them" is comparatively easy to draw. But gay women and men are the children of everybody else: the sons and daughters of Vaucluse, Carlton, Moonee Valley, Thursday Island—everywhere. And if the statistics are correct, it is not mere homosexuality which is the basis of their gay identity. More homosexual acts take place in apparently heterosexual contexts than in gay-defined ones.

So where do we draw the line around this community? I don't know; neither do the sociologists. But we do know that so-called "straight" men especially go to great extremes to make sure there is no confusion. The greatest insult you can pay a "real" Australian male is to mistake him for gay. This is why the collapse of the boundaries at the end of the Mardi Gras parade (Act 1) is such a radical moment. A totally "mixed" crowd surges across that cherished line between straight and gay and for an hour or two takes over the streets of Darlinghurst and Surry Hills, actors in a drama of liberation our society rarely permits.

The consequences are not so dramatic as this might imply. No orgies in the streets, as in San Francisco; no public sex, as in Rio; not even any great violence (by contrast, the death rate for Rio's Mardi Gras averaged 37 per day this year). But there was a struggle for territory, to redefine the streets of inner Sydney, that continued for hours. The result was not licentious, but *communitas*—for everybody, gay, straight, or whatever (this last probably the largest category). All that dreadfully heavy gender baggage dropped, if only for an hour or two.

Down in Moore Park, and around the Showground, spontaneous dramas were played out. A couple of fellows stomped a bus shelter to death in an ecstatic breakdance on the roof, generating their own disco sound effects and attracting a crowd. Around the Showground, people unwilling to pay the entry fees simply danced the night away outside at their own spontaneous, unofficial party. Small knots of people of every description assembled on street corners from the Cross to Paddington and down through Surry Hills. Electricity was tangible, well into the morning.

Around midnight, the police moved back onto Oxford Street to reclaim possession of the streets with the aid of the big council sweeping machines. They were not undisputed. Thousands of revelers remained in the area and were loathe to relinquish their new territory and its freedoms. That took another hour, and a great deal of shouting and broken glass. The first line of ill-advised private autos came through dodging a sea of bodies and a carpet of chiffon, tinnies, and glitter.

This was when the party teetered most delicately on the political, and it became possible to understand how uprisings and revolutions begin at such moments. Here, not at the wild but contained party in the Showground, the real potential of Sydney's Gay Mardi Gras in the coming years could be glimpsed. It was as close as I want to get to the "Day of the Locust." And it suggests that if Mardi Gras continues to grow at its annual increment, both the city and the organizers will have to rethink the event. The capacity of the forces of order to reclaim the streets, and the night, seemed barely adequate, and perhaps not entirely necessary. Next year, why not leave Oxford Street blocked off until morning?

I haven't considered the Mardi Gras Festival week, the official calendar of sports tournaments, openings, film and theater events provided by the Mardi Gras Association, which extends the festival over a full month. The shameful fact is that I missed even those events I had booked to attend. There always seemed to be something else going on—another party, a different (unscheduled) film, an interstate friend to catch up with.

Maybe there's a lesson here, too. The festival calendar itself seemed disappointing. Too many imported overseas acts, for example. Too little representation of Sydney's own dynamic arts and criticism scene (which grew up through the gay movement and its press in the 1970s but was oddly excluded from participation).

In fact, many more arguably "gay" arts could be seen off the schedule than on. Ethyl Eichelberger had just finished an amazing season at the Belvoir Street Theatre, a production of Genet's *The Maids* was at the City Acting Studio, and one could also see *Vampire Lesbians of Sodom*, Frank Chickens, not to mention all the usual campy and kitschy opera and ballet seasons around, all of which, if not strictly gay, invoke aspects of gender criticism and gay sources. It was also a very rich period for film. The excellent Spanish genderfuck film *Law of Desire* was at the Dendy, Frank Moorhouse's peculiar *Everlasting Secret Family* opened at the Academy, and gay characters and gender themes featured in a half dozen other mainstream and imported films available that week.

By comparison, the official arts schedule actually verged on cultural cringe, and seemed more derivative of overseas definitions of gayness than we require now. It was not improved by having American critic

Vito Russo return to "replay" his *Celluloid Closet* lecture, which seems uninformed in contrast to the sophisticated criticism of *Filmnews* and the Sydney criticism scene.

My point is simple: the Sydney Mardi Gras does not succeed at delineating a community, nor should it try. Our community is Sydney itself. Maybe it is not so far-fetched for gay people to consider the analogy to the medieval guilds, collectivities of craft, residence, and ideology which staged the original Carnivales.

Modern Mardi Gras now articulates the interdependence of the gay world with all other local scenes. It breaks down the boundaries, and liberates us all when this happens. This is, in 1988, a political act with radical potential. By contrast, the narrowly defined, even cliquish "gay" events of the festival seemed comparatively trivial when contrasted to the parade itself, and the spontaneous street theater that followed.

The organizers deserve maximum credit, not only for hard work, but for managing this impossibly complex and elaborate event so well. Yet the Sydney Gay Mardi Gras this year also showed its capacity to grow organically, unofficially, beyond its committees, its schedules, its intentions, into—for one night only—the biggest and best show in town.

March 20, 1988

Perhaps by selecting out only what seem to me the high points of a day or week to report here, I misrepresent my actual daily life considerably. But instead of depicting a dashing whirlwind of engaged activity, my most exciting moments, in combination, are likely to seem so trivial that they'll convey to any reader something less than a notable existence, which seems to me to be the case. It might be even more accurate to write down the recipe I worked out for chicken pie today, to describe the time and difficulty that cooking and eating poses for me each day. There's no getting around the Bhagavadgita admonition: "He who cooks for himself eats sin." And yet, what's on offer in the local takeaways is something worse than sin. So I cook, and eat, as I do almost everything, by myself. Maybe I should also admit how much TV I watch now, and how, for example, I was recently addicted to certain American sitcoms of no conceivable worth (only their very familiarity appealed, especially the opportunity to see black and Jewish women's humor). I refuse completely to watch Australian drama or comedy series, but do watch news, current affairs, and some documentaries. And I remain addicted to local and national talk shows. That's three or four hours a day. I piss a lot, shit once a day, jerk off maybe once a week, and spend a lot of time on long-distance phone calls. Monday and Tuesday, I teach my tutes, and go in to school at least one other day a week.

Reading fiction, oddly, seems even more of an indulgence. I'm currently finishing [Guy Hocquenghem's] *Love in Relief*, which John sent (why? I asked him, and accused him of not knowing how else to get rid of it, but it turns out to be even more peculiar than it first seemed and something intriguing about its objectifications continues to engage me). I put down that awful book about picture making in the Amazon in the last chapters. It was simply too offensive. It's not as easy as it might seem to find entertaining books which don't prove insultingly dumb.

Took myself to see *The Last Emperor* around the corner today—fully $8's worth of movie. In fact, the wonderfully rich visual detail (and the extreme exotica of the first 15 minutes) were equal, momentarily, to my hunger for high art. So what if its politics stank and its ethics were overmanipulated ambiguities. The scenes in the Forbidden City brought me back to the Oriental Rooms of the Philadelphia Museum. I now actually think it was better to grow up there than it would have been to grow up near the Metropolitan. The scale of the Philly is so much better for a kid; it's comparatively finite, and so locatable in the world in the way the Metropolitan (or the Louvre, or the Hermitage) refuses because it takes over the world. I wonder about arranging to get a Yuendumu painting donated. I find myself returning to scenes of childhood more often, piecing together bits of events I'm surprised my memory still contains.

Athol says Warwick fucked up my salary increase on the secondment. Bloody shit; I need that extra money to get out of here. Athol's furious because he, and his brief in this, were contravened. Dear Lord, can't anything go smoothly? Not even worth describing the immigration business. John called Friday to say he and Liz were going to arrange my life for me, but as it turned out, I'd already gone to work on most of the aspects they'd thought through. I said if my plans fall through, they can pick up the pieces if they want. I'll be too buggered to.

March 29, 1988

A week without entries—a sure sign something's up. But not especially. Penny came up Thursday; she had to go up to Cherbourg (how French that sounds—perhaps we'll ski!) for the weekend to check pictures and captions for the book [*After 200 Years: Photographic Essays of Aboriginal and Islander Australia Today*]. Odd, this book. It has a very powerful existence though it doesn't yet exist, which may be unhealthy. My own book [*For a Cultural Future: Francis Jupurrurla Makes TV at Yuendumu*] came from Juan yesterday, and I can still barely look at it. Every flaw (mostly slack citations) wags at me like an accusing finger. I rush by sentences which seem too dense for sense on first reading instead of checking to see if they do make any sense. Thursday and Friday, Adrian Martin was here with his girlfriend to use my computer to finish editing *Photofile*. He was not very communicative, although at some point Penny got him talking. Maybe he's shy. The sum effect was that it got very busy around here, so I promptly ran a high fever and took to bed. In fact, I became rather worried about myself.

Dr. K. has had to write all these letters describing my health for various bureaucratic audiences (immigration, parking permits, etc.). These are very tragic documents: they describe me as having terminal cancer, anaemia, TB, or whatever will be most convincing to the recipient. And I do have all these things, though only one per letter. I feel odd, but not disinterested, handing these over the counter and watching people read them. They get very polite. I suppose I would, too. I cannot quite grasp what it must seem to people to see me around in the usual places and the usual way, but know I am more intimate with death than is permitted. But am I? It's all gotten very abstract again. In fact, the Kaposi's (those little circlets of morbidity) mainly are what remind me of my condition. Otherwise, I'd only feel somewhat weak, and not very much at that. But I do wonder what happens next. I maintain a sort of plateau; only the cancer is progressive. Nasty, ugly, but not physically disabling. What then should I expect to come down the pike and knock me off my chair? I suppose I'm superstitious now that the book's finally out.

April 3, 1988

Look a gift horse in the mouth! I've been ragged and paranoid all week. Fevers and sweats coming and going and some odd lung thing that's scary. My tumors itch and seem to be developing psoriatic complications or something. It's been raining as long as I can recall; everything is mold, mold, mold. The kitchen is filled with flying weevils. The toilet is backed up. My neighbor has taken up the saxophone and tries to play hits from *The Sound of Music* all day. I can't sleep and can't do anything but. I wake up repeatedly in the middle of the night with the horrors. I don't even want to call anybody. I have no interest in working and I haven't even been pursuing my immigration business responsibly. My physician seems to have deserted me. My conviction that the world I perceive corresponds to anybody else's is slipping. Maybe I died in November and this is some awful postmortem fantasy I inhabit now?

Went to the cheap bookstore and stocked up on mostly gay novels. These turned out to be mostly terrible, terrible. Mills & Boon for poofters. So depressing. Even worse than TV, which is again completely unwatchable. Did go to see *Cane Toads* with Lee and Stuart and Jo and Gillian and Leda (the follow-through of a dinner the previous evening at Stuart's). Why am I so committed to non-mass media? Why am I so determined to remain in poverty, a victim? When will it ever stop raining?

April 9, 1988

The Aboriginal Institute's executive committee met at Griffith Friday, preceded by a supper Thursday night. I dolled up and went, and then joined them for lunch Friday. What an odd assortment. I'm getting much more comfortably casual about what really is a highly calculated and constrained politics of discourse. When Warwick tried to talk to me about my salary (as though by having the balls to do so, he secures my consent) I simply changed the subject to something more casual, like the cricket, and prattled on. Nic and Bob T. were a bit more probing; they both wanted to talk about the Chatwin book (and Nic wanted to know about mine). So we did. It has become a set piece. I buy my way into the good old boys' conversation with insider knowledge, which now includes Annette's infinitely more clever Chatwin piece, which she just sent me. I'm so terribly uncomfortable with all this. Nobody wanted to talk about Sally Morgan's book [*My Place*], since they all just loved it. That's why it's good to have reviewed a popular and unpopular (at least in my crowd) book together, and claimed they say the same thing. And why I'll have to reject *Oceania*'s offer to publish my review [of Chatwin's and Morgan's books] only if I break it into two.

But I've been under this awful weather now for weeks, still running a fever sort of randomly, sometimes quite high, and all kinds of strange other symptoms. Dr. K.'s off in New York and London, so I'm semi-deserted. I'm having trouble sleeping nights, and none sleeping days, which is all I really want to do. And it makes me quite crazy and obsessed in the head.

Read the dreadful biography of dreadful Edie Sedgwick, and recalled what schizophrenia was in the hip late 1960s. And how young women especially tried to emulate a certain style of psychosis, and sometimes succeeded. The book does mount a good case for judging Warhol an evil monster, even if it fails to pinpoint precisely how responsibility is to be assessed in the curious universe he created with such apparent passive ease. Interesting to have confirmed that blacks were excluded from that world, so that in my own (and probably many other teenies') case, I was trying to play to what may have been opposed, or exclusive, domains of hip: Warhol's disinterested chic and get-down motherfucker soul at the same time.

April 11, 1988

No, it will never stop raining. It has now exceeded all historical records for April rainfall. Michael from QuAC came in to clean today (he is miraculously reliable) and poured bleach all over everything, relieving me from the omnipresent mold, and imparting a nice cleanly chemical smell. I went out and bought bug spray and tried to reduce the weevil population. Stuff the ozone layer!

What's been keeping me up the last few nights has been this bizarre five-page (single-spaced) letter the Santa Theresa Catholic Aboriginal community sent to Minister Hand, petitioning for increased funding for broadcasting development for their community (at least, I think that's what it's asking for—each time I read it, I come out with a different impression). They spend much of the letter attributing their problems to me, in a variety of very convoluted ways, which somehow assumes that I drafted all current government policy. All this out of a pleasant daytrip to the community with Freda and Francis in 1984! They also claim that I snuck into the community that time without permission, and failed to speak with any of their officials or senior members of the community, both of which are simply lies. After I read this thing, the realization came over me (rather like Rita Tushingham in *The Knack*, on discovering she'd been raped) that I had been slandered, in precisely those terms the law describes. An odd feeling. But who wants to take a Catholic priest and an Aboriginal community to court? I've written Freda, noting that CAAMA [Central Australian Aboriginal Media Association] took me out there, did broker a permit through their council for me, and took responsibility then, and so should consider if they can find a way to work this out. And I wrote to Dr. Coombs via Nancy because this thing will hit Hand's desk at just about the same time as my immigration appeal. These bloody cretins seeking a few thousand extra bucks really could wreck me beyond what they ever imagine! But then, they seem to have whipped themselves up into a considerable frenzy about me, and they make me sound like some kind of white debil-debil manipulating blackfellas throughout the Centre. How could they have harbored all this without me ever having an inkling? As I say, bizarre. At least when I can't get back to sleep at three in the morning, I have something to do—drafting imaginary replies.

Athol called to say the executive restored my full salary. I deserve no less for having behaved myself for maybe the first such time ever!

April 14, 1988

If I continue to live much longer, I will have to learn to read French, speak Warlpiri, and spell English. There are arguments both ways.

April 17, 1988

I still feel wretched. But then, this is the longest period I've remained in Brisbane for some time. And it's been awful. My flat is noisier than ever, my attempts to complain only make my neighbors think I'm crazy and evil. It's nasty and bizarre. It becomes hard to judge how much of my feeling awful is connected to how awful life at home is and how crazy, bored, stressed, and psychotic I've been. I had to drag myself out to the Queensland Art Gallery to look at the Aboriginal show. Though I lasted less than an hour before wearying, it did improve my day and my outlook, if not the cramps in my stomach (new symptom—probably the result of my crazy cooking). I need to see how I'll manage my trips to Sydney and Melbourne over the next few weeks, and how much I'll need to protect myself: hotels or whatever, schedules, etc. It may be that my condition has slipped another notch, but I'll wait till Dr. K. returns to discuss that.

My lovely lawyer called Thursday to say that the local immigration office will recommend me for a year's extension on my working visa. A year, I think, would be quite sufficient. I'm not ready to take a deep breath yet (having been through this before). I am also cautious about the possibility of a trick; they want me to give up my backup request for resident status, which would leave me totally unprotected if the recommendation doesn't go through.

April 19, 1988

Off to Sydney tomorrow for the launch [of *For A Cultural Future*], video showing, and general public displays. I've mixed feelings about this, its purpose and benefits, not to mention my own ability to sustain the energy—and the masque—required. I'd almost just as soon simply visit friends for a week. But it seems helpful to keep myself visibly interesting, and interested. Something will have to pull me out of this morose ennui, and it's unlikely to happen in Brisbane.

I've been working on another Aboriginal art essay, explaining the last two. Except as a form of therapy, I again don't know what the purpose is (although I'll need something to read in Melbourne and elsewhere next month; it seems one has to keep producing these things in order to get around). I am also seeking a grammar and a poetics that will let me render things more clearly. I'm still very tentative about the monograph, and unsure if I actually believe that modern criticism must be difficult to read to respect its own problematizations and to keep the reader on her toes. I do seem marginally better the last few days. Working does seem to help. My home life has gotten so obsessional—too much like my crazy mother's.

Went to hear Aboriginal poet Colin Johnson [Mudrooroo] at U.Q. today. Très postmoderne, utterly disconnected, and rather fun. A relief, as I'd like to talk with him, publicly as well as privately. Did get into a rave with Koories from the local media association, and realized I know a good deal that could be useful to them. But do I have the motivation, let alone the stamina, to get involved in another "Birth of the Station"? What is nice is that it was a comfortable and familiar chat, no confrontative bullshit; we both acknowledged we knew what we were talking about, I guess. But what strikes me again and again is that I really do like Aborigines—though that's too racist and imprecise, put that way. But they are engaged, in a way that white Australians tend not to be. Their circumstances are interesting, to them and me. They tend to be kind. And no matter how hard they try, they mostly fail to be bourgeois. They are too familiar with poverty and suffering perhaps. I feel a whole lot less self-conscious about the way I look and my visible marks of disease when I'm with blacks. They seem a good deal less concerned.

April 26, 1988

The book launch was wonderful, but scary, because it came unnervingly close to "my perfect guest list." As John had anticipated, it would have made a wonderful party without bothering with showing the videos. Those videos did give me indigestion, and worse. A complete nightmare: half of what was promised didn't come through, people calling the airlines and freight offices till the last minute. . . . Bloody awful pain I could have done without. Still, it was worth showing the stuff, even under the execrable conditions of the Chauvel screen. I did apologize to the paying audience. They may have taken it all as further evidence of authenticity. But also, I was able to appear active and in full stride rather than being carted in on a stretcher.

The whole trip was really an awful effort. There were some fine occasions I couldn't quite rise to, and opportunities for socializing I didn't quite connect to. One of those efforts whose pleasures are delayed—perhaps like tourism? Surely a day spent at the new, and inhuman, Brisbane airport due to strikes in Sydney, getting misinformed, misdirected, and shuttled on and off planes like baggage didn't help. Then to return home (my little layer cake of agro) so I can go through it all again next day! An inauspicious start, at best.

And then dear Paul, who seems partly recovered from his physical ills, praise God, seemed to be wallowing in some mental ones. At John's dinner, he was very testy, very critical of me and my work, not perhaps undeservedly so. It wasn't merely or even: "I made you and I can break you." But something else. I noticed a number of people leaning on me in odd ways all weekend. Except John, who was grand, but who explains all these things via what is for me a too-easy psychologizing (though in John's hands, it's really quite complex). Paul settled down after we had a private chat, me deferring (as I think is warranted). But then at the launch, he and Juan disappeared early without a word, and didn't join us for dinner as planned. Well, I am beyond worrying a great deal about these things, but something's going on, and some feelings seem to be on some line. Surely, it's an odd experience to be feted in the Sydney arts and intellectual scenes. And perhaps I was, fortunately, somewhat too concerned just getting through the physical requirements to make a great deal of that fact. But if indeed Marcia's incredibly laudatory launch speech is published, and when some of the reviews come out, I'll be subjected to another version of that. Modesty is neither an adequate nor popular response to all this.

Maybe the nicest part (at risk of insulting a considerable number of people who worked their butts off for me) was Friday's trip to the Hermitage exhibit at the Art Gallery of New South Wales. A number of lovely pieces, some very surprising if you imagine you know their author or period. The penultimate room, delicious! A fabulous, radical Matisse; a very peculiar, good Manet; a surprise Cézanne and an expected one. I like small exhibits! And I love luscious oil paint.

April 27, 1988

Odd dreams. I am in bed, a fairly Chekhovian setting, attended by two women: the mother and the sister (not ones I have, or even remember having met—still, they are "mine"). From bed, I direct the building of something which, in the next episode, turns out to be a chapel: lovely light wood of traditional construction, small, even cozy, truncated naves, unornamented, and windows that seem to open out onto woods, rocks and trees. Only I can't see out much from my vantage point in the central area (altar?) where my bed is, and the two women and I casually chat—about what? I can't remember.

Why such obvious Bergman mise-en-scène? Why so Christian? This coffin, a premonition of death? I'm not convinced, although I returned from Sydney sick as a dog, barely able to board the plane, and feared I'd land straight away in hospital. Perhaps death is not such an odd dream to have on such a fevered night. And why women? In fact, I also dreamed of first love Stephanie, a completely seductive dream, she poised as *La maja desnuda*. I started with her breast, but didn't really get much further than comfort; little sex.

I did look at my cock today and find (without difficulty) the lesion I knew would be there. My last domain succumbs; no named extremity, limb, or body part remains unulcerated now. I take some perverse pride that my cock should succumb last.

May 1, 1988

Spent the weekend in hospital getting "topped up." My hemoglobin had fallen dreadfully. No wonder I couldn't get up the stairs and had trouble sleeping; bad dreams. Odd that I shouldn't have recognized this was the problem, only it now isn't the only one. It's hard to separate out symptoms. I did not bound from bed fully restored this morning, I'm afraid. (Never quite like the first time!) Still a variety of nasty, uncomfortable symptoms: throat, chest, belly, skin, fevers.

Richard suggested interferon. It seems the KS may be responsible for some internal blocking or irritation that is making me feel lousy. Or maybe it's CMV thingies swimming around in my blood. We can only hypothesize, and then balance out the various risks. Interferon, for example, may remit the cancer, but reduce further my T-cells and assure increasing opportunistic infections. And so it goes. I said, why bother? He said, we'll talk about it after you're topped up. So we went for brunch today, but talked about the Hockney and Mapplethorpe exhibits he's seen on his overseas trip. And about staying in the Australian U.N. mission guest flat, formerly Oscar Hammerstein's apartment on Fifth and 87th. Really, all I want is something comfy with a good outlook to retire to myself. Not so easy.

Whatever fantasies I had of going into hospital so that I could relax and people could take care of me have again been disabused. The transfusion was not fun, people were not efficient, and the food was even more awful than I'd talked myself out of remembering. The usual string of procedural bizarreries. My favorite was when the head nurse came in around 10:30 last night to announce that they had no instructions to remove the needle in my arm (only to insert it and pump blood through for 16 hours). Would I authorize the removal and relieve them of legal responsibility? Rather like being given permission to jump up in the air, but not to come down! My sarcasm, largely restrained until then, flooded the room and swept the entire nursing staff into the hall.

May 6, 1988

I'm supposed to be in Melbourne, fabulous Melbourne, pronouncing on the state of Australian art and criticism at a prestige intellectual forum. Instead, I'm still in Brisbane, banal, horrid Brisbane, lying in bed and sweating. My fevers are recurrent, my energy limited, and my mood morose. This is the first commitment I can think of that I've missed because of my illness, and I'm perhaps more devastated than is strictly justified. But it's been a rough week to drag myself through, and the cumulative effect of the fevers is a kind of surreal disorientation. I did get a paper written and faxed off, and dear Ross will read it for me, although it reflects my mental confusion, and, I fear, isn't very good. Even so, I will look at least minimally responsible, I hope. Richard wanted to put me in hospital for a week. I quite panicked and we compromised on an elaborate course of pills—by next week I'll have a daily intake of about thirty pills, seven or eight varieties. This is an attempt to improve my quality of life. I'm not entirely convinced.

Obviously, I haven't done much this week. Read through two Isherwood books. The earlier one (*Lions and Shadows*) was pretty thin, although the portraits of Cambridge life fascinate me—such an expensive cultural infrastructure propping up an educational institution! We here in Australia are stripping all universities down to the bare bones right now (and only the profitable bones at that) and then financially penalizing the students for having the cheek to want to study. But my interest in Cambridge is more personal. It describes the world I fantasized would become mine when I became an academic and now discover is further away than ever, maybe in time as well as space. *Down There on a Visit* was much more fun, as Isherwood is writing well here, and is so accessible, even familiar, somehow. To a literate, academic faggot like myself, he is very close to home. Yet repeatedly, especially when he describes his relations to his current guru (as in other books), something goes quite sour for me. I am not hostile to those people, or those disciplines, though I suspect it made a lot of difference in my life to have encountered their equivalent in my youth, and in the cultural moment of the 1960s and 1970s. But what leaks through his prose at that point is a suspicion that there is some massive self-deception, some basis in sexual/gender guilt at work in Isherwood's case that remains totally opaque to him. Even his earlier relationships: Waldemar is depicted as selfish, stupid and unattractive in all ways but the physical, a traitor to whatever sexuality he may himself express. What is the basis of the bond there? While I make it a rule never to judge my own friends' taste in sexual/romantic objects, I do think it difficult to justify how Isherwood's obsessive reflexivity stops abruptly when considering his own desires. It was the 1950s, though, and so *Down There* must be acknowledged as a courageous book, seminal in gay literature and politics. But now we need descriptions of our promiscuity, the desire which drove us out as hunters, which expressed itself in certain preferences and acts. I hate to think that deluded old egotist John Rechy will in the end prove our best chronicler.

Richard says that two-thirds of AB-positives are still healthy after seven years. That's encouraging news, along with the statistic that almost no new positives are being reported in San Francisco. I wonder all over again if I could have avoided this somehow. Never did get over my conviction that I would follow Rick to the grave. Not that I believe so much in the power of positive thinking here, nor, more importantly, that I would have abandoned my life (and work) to save my life. Still, my fatalism may not have been helpful. The only thing I would have considered doing differently would have been to quit Griffith and abandon Queensland as soon as I saw what a mess it was here. But that would have only propelled me into a different, and equally stressful, mess at that point. There never really do seem to be any alternatives.

May 22, 1988

Kings Cross

Dear John

A densely strange week, perhaps hypnotically so. I spent much of it on my back, as I'm sorry to say I slipped another notch, especially in terms of energy. But the psychological trauma of my father and Mitzi (new stepmother) surely was draining in its own right.

Liz helped the first two days. Eventually I snapped at her and she disappeared. Then Dr. Richard flew in and that was the next night's dinner. And Penny came in for 36 hours Friday–Saturday (she seems miraculously calmer and really improved).

It was very difficult with Dad. I'm appalled at how much Oedipal shit I dredged up—how much resentment I discovered and how I handled it like a six-year-old. I was very uncomfortable with Mitzi, though I withhold judgment; what a spot she must have felt she was in! It took till Saturday to get my father away, alone, to spend some time in an intimate discussion without her running interference (his doing, I suspect, more than hers). But going back to Cape Cod no longer seems like a very attractive idea.

Paul called. I keep forgetting how terrified he is of disease and medicine. I realize he's been very brave in my case. He says the Centre Georges Pompidou wants to translate me into French! And Juan tells me some of my stuff is circulating in Spanish. Tom O'Regan replied very responsibly to my letter and called me here. I've left open the decisions on what form his critical collection [in *Continuum*] should take for now. And Paul, out of the blue, resurrected the idea of an essay collection. I hope I will be forgiven if I express a somewhat distanced interest in all that, however, as I am more concerned that I may be reaching a point where it will be difficult to care for myself, and am more involved in that problem.

I spoke with a counselor from the Ankali Foundation—wonderful, no bullshit, an informed, helpful lady. That already makes a difference. I will still try to relocate from here to Sydney unless I'm even further gone than we suspect, although some details remain vague. With my father's help, I'm now able to commit $1,200–$1,500 per month for a flat. That should do it!

Which reminds me: Ann punked out on your deal and rented her flat. So, no go. She said she'd call you.

Gavin, who has some spare time since the Powerhouse train took off, offered to do the flat hunting for me. I think he actually could succeed, so I'll leave that with him.

Sorry your flat isn't in quite as terrific shape as you left it, but cleaning is a bit rough for me. I do hope everything's in order. The bedspread is a present.

Now that the second construction (or deconstruction) site is underway out front, it has become clear that what they've been doing out there for the past year is distilling the most perfectly annoying cacophony—the ultimately irritating noise. I now actually find it most interesting. The addition of the whistle is, I think, a masterstroke. Poor dear; I now see at least one good reason for your Fiji trip.

So you absolutely will/must get to Brisbane on June 6 as you planned. We can luxuriate in the far less dramatic sounds of small industry above and punk rock from below. I do hope to be able to spend some chat time together soon.

Love, etc.

May 25, 1988

New Farm

Dear Gavin

Gore Vidal on TV the other night showed us Henry James's rooms in some American millionaire's palace in Venice. I thought that would do very nicely, but in case you missed the program, here are some thoughts, preferences, and requirements I have for lodging in Sydney.

What I'm looking for is most succinctly described as a quiet flat of indeterminate size (anywhere from a very spacious bedsitter to a three-bedroom flat—each size has its advantages), located in an indeterminate but probably Eastern suburb, conveniently sited, easy access, partly or fully furnished, with an exterior view, via balcony or garden.

There surely are elements of fantasy as well as unrealistic expectations in my thinking about all this. Admitting this, allow me to elaborate the main criteria, not as a set of determinate rules, but so as to let you in on that fantasy and put you in a better position to make a choice among what really does turn out to be available for the $300–$350 per week I can pay.

AESTHETICS: My first considerations (practical or not) really are aesthetic. I'm likely to be house-bound much of the time, and in a reclining position for a good deal of any day. The bedroom will be important, and probably a second (lounge?) room also to recline in, perhaps where a desk can be as well. Think of any flat you might see from this relatively immobilized perspective. That main room needs somehow to resist claustrophobia. French windows, balconies, gardens and other interesting access and outlooks would be most desirable, perhaps even more from the bedroom than the lounge. Anything interesting (sea, city, harbor, birds, trees) to look out on would be a blessing.

PRIVACY: Equally important is peace and quiet. No major construction within 150 meters, no obviously noisy neighbors, good sound insulation, and reasonable visual seclusion. It's noise that's driving me out of Brisbane more than anything, but I realize this is a difficult matter to ascertain casually. Construction may rule out the Cross and Potts Point, for example, otherwise very desirable neighborhoods.

SIZE: I'm not terribly fussed about the number of rooms. Two generous-sized rooms, plus kitchen and bath, could do. More might be nice; if large enough, I could look for a flatmate, an idea which has some attractions. But both kitchen and bath should be simple, modern, and easily cleaned. Bathroom must have a full bath.

FURNISHINGS: Ideally, the flat would be at least partly furnished. Merely built-ins, appliances, and a lounge suite might be sufficient. I don't imagine I can really afford to worry much about this, but a horribly cluttered kitschy interior would be out of the question. Simple and modern would be preferable. I'd consider minimal furniture, but good stove, refrigerator, and a washer/dryer (or access to one) are essential.

LOCATION: I don't have a suburb absolutely in mind. The convenience of the Cross, Potts Point, and Elizabeth Bay are appealing. It would be especially good to be able to walk to shops, transport, easily. But these tend to be noisy suburbs. Darlinghurst and Paddington are feasible, especially if near Oxford Street. But I have a sense that flats tend to be claustrophobic around there. Bondi: difficult, but then for an ocean view . . . Double Bay, Rose Bay, Edgecliff, Woollahra—all could be possible (again, for the views) but seem a bit difficult in terms of shops and transport. Centennial Park?

A real problem may well prove that I can't do extended inclines. No more than a reasonable flight of stairs to the flat—preferably none—or a lift. And, for example, much of Elizabeth Bay would be out because the streets are too hilly for me.

That's most of it. I can't believe that you (or anyone, actually) would take on such a chore for anybody less than blood kin (and perhaps especially not them). So it's especially difficult to express my appreciation for your even attempting this. I hope that if I do make this move successfully, you also will enjoy my being in Sydney, so that some mutual advantage is gained here. Thanks again.

Regards, etc.

May 26, 1988

My face itches.

This actually is subjectively my most annoying symptom at the moment, although I am spectacularly weak suddenly, and I don't know why. Dr. K. took blood yesterday. But it's all such a game of probabilities; so many things are floating around my system, it's probably impossible to sort out what's causing what with any precision. What AZT seems to do is keep you alive so that you can become host to an increasing array of exotic and even novel malaises. He took me off one of my medications on the hypothesis that that was responsible for my weakness, appetite loss, nausea, and general ill health. But what's odd is that if I just lay in bed, only my itchy face is bothersome.

I am a bit frightened because this really is below the level of functioning that allows me to care for myself. I mean, I really can't manage alone with this little energy. And it reminds me that nobody else is going to take care of me either, and sends me off into a meditation about how this extraordinary situation has come to be: partly a result of choices I've made, equally a consequence of circumstances. I remember when I was quite young thinking that the very worst thing would be to end up as an old fart with pee-stained underwear. So I stopped wearing underwear.

May 27, 1988

I didn't make it to the Queensland Institute of Technology communications conference: fascist, blue-sky technocrats vs. screw-you-whitefella do-nothing black activists, I'd guess. It would take considerable stamina to get through that. But Liz came up, and in the evening dragged Freda over for a visit. What a wonderful time we had. After Liz left for her plane, Freda and I went to dinner, and talked a mile a minute. She said she'd cried all the way over on the plane from Alice

Springs because she knew she would see me and thought she'd find me on death's door. I did the best I could to be reassuring, but physically the evening was a bit rough for me. After she left, I threw up a $20 steak.

It's not easy to define my friendship with Freda. The politics are very difficult. But the affection is immense, and at the level of chat and gossip, we have such a fine time.

May 28, 1988

One of those desperate, dismal Saturdays. Yesterday, my landlord called to say I'd forgotten the rent. I said I was ill and it would take some doing to get someone to the bank for me. I'd arrange it first thing next week. Today, they called back and demanded immediate payment or they'd serve an eviction notice. I went totally berserk on the phone. I really haven't slipped into that mode in some time. But I got right into it. I had to call around to find somebody to intercede for me. Nobody was home; Jo finally responded to the message I left on Stuart's machine, called them, and made the arrangements.

This put me into the bleakest mood; not that soon I couldn't care for myself, but that already I couldn't. Moving to Sydney, or anywhere, seems completely unrealistic. I can barely make it from my bed to the bathroom! I spent part of the day fantasizing suicide/funeral arrangements, but couldn't get very far with the logistics here either. Anyway, how much does it matter? I assert that I am unlocated, that I relate to no particular place, a radical inversion of both Zionism and Aboriginal philosophy. Place of death—inconsequential. Cremation appropriate; scatter my ashes to the wind, perhaps on a seashore somewhere, invoking air, fire, land, and water simultaneously, and proving that I always pathologically avoided making choices. But having said this, what right do I have to be so insistent that I not end in Brisbane? If I refuse any identification with place, how can I single out a place for exclusion. Or maybe more to the point, why not just give it all up? What makes me think I have to stage-manage this as well? I'm sure death itself is the simplest thing in the world. The choice seems merely to be this: to arrange everything, to maintain a morbid fantasy of control, or simply give it up and let it go. The latter looks more and more appealing.

June 6, 1988

I called Richard and arranged to see him at 8 A.M. My energy is completely gone. The slightest effort has me panting desperately and violently headachey.

In his office I said, "It's getting nasty now. Can you get me out of this?" We both cried a bit, and he arranged to check me into hospital. I drove my car home, waited for the QuAC cleaner, told her what was happening. She straightened up, cleaned out the fridge, and so forth. I packed and grabbed a taxi to Wattlebrae. I reckoned I had a few days left, at best (or worst), and wasn't displeased with the timing, felt reasonably resolved, even satisfied. I would try to get Athol to print out the journal and get it to Paul. The letter to Gavin would be a good place to duck out, even.

June 15, 1988

But you don't die, at least right away. This is AIDS, the disease of a thousand rehearsals. After a few days, Richard succeeded in making me reasonably comfortable. I read some more I. B. Singer. Michael from QuAC, Stuart, and assorted Griffithites visited intermittently. Had the usual fights with the doctors, the staff, and the dietitian. My condition didn't seem to improve; in fact, my KS was swelling and uncomfortable and ugly.

I spend considerable time trying to figure out what possible point there is to drawing this out any further. But as I'm not really in pain, it also seems a bit unsporting to terminate, mostly out of boredom. They've sent the hospital psychiatrist over, presumably to discuss this, though it's hard to tell with shrinks just what they're there for. Such an odd, faux-dialogue. Anyway, John, Paul, Penny, and even brother Mark have scheduled visits, and I suppose that I should hang out for those and maybe even try to finish up some writing if I can motivate myself at all.

June 16, 1988

I'm in a Mexican prison actually, and with no relatives in town to call on. My only hope is to bribe the guards or pass a letter through the window. They feed us the leftovers from last night for breakfast, lunch, and even dinner—mince eternally reformed. Mostly, they call it savory meatballs. I'd surrender my life (and divulge all my secrets) for a chocolate ice-cream cone (as it does seem a bit late in the game for health foods).

June 19, 1988

John is here. What a relief. We talk.

Treating my weakness as an adrenal virus with cortisone supplements has increased my strength unbelievably. We've gone for rides, and today even went for lunch at the Grandview Hotel on Cleveland Bay. A miracle! I toy with the idea that there may yet be a month-or-more's reprieve, but have decided there's no psychological advantage and little evidential reason for doing so. Still, I'm much more chipper, and have started writing again. Nearly finished the Aboriginal appropriation art piece for the IMA. Remarkably, it's fairly good/interesting.

June 20, 1988

Wattlebrae

Dear Gavin

What a lovely, and brave letter. Thanks so for it. I hope this reply doesn't seem too macabre. Obviously, you weren't expecting one. But I thought I'd let you know I'm hanging on yet. The characteristic of this disease is that every phase seems to be drawn out and out, and every crisis has a hundred rehearsals. One purpose of this letter is to reassure you that the disease remains very kind to me. I remain lucid (indeed, I've got my laptop here and continue to edit and revise some articles) and only minimally uncomfortable. The hardest part really is maintaining resistance to the institutional discourses of the public hospital system so as to retain some dignity, assurance, and self-definition. Friends visiting have contributed greatly to that. All this despite the fact that I really am headed for the last round-up. My blood is nearly water and nothing stands between me and a thousand exotic bacteria and infections, any of which could turn me belly-up in no time.

And to let you know that Foss plans to get my journals of the last ten months into publication quickly, and you might find those interesting.

I had planned to end them with a letter I wrote you but never sent (days before I returned to hospital), describing a fantasy of an apartment (and a life) I wanted to live in Sydney which you so generously had offered to help me find. I thought the letter offered a poignant fake closure to the journal, but now I suppose it must be superseded by the somewhat less symmetrical facts of the last few weeks. Be brave and take care.

Love, etc.

June 21, 1988

John and I stayed up till 1 A.M. with the tape recorder. I thought we'd tackle some esoterica about my work and writing, the intersections of our politics, etc. But instead, he solicited a life history. In two hours of tape, we only got from 1969 to 1972, and only from New Mexico to New York (via Boston). Valium turns out to be a wonderful fuel for the mouth, and I thoroughly enjoyed the rap. Curious contrast to the unsatisfying monologue for the shrink. My account for John was also full of set pieces (these years have become an iconicized moment, of course, and we who manned the cultural barricades have a responsibility for the artfulness of our storytelling). So it wasn't quite a dialogue, but John commented and remembered too, and where he directed questioning it was often in reference to other talks we had and issues that I or he have maintained an interest in (such as the creative monsters—Warhol, Fassbinder, etc.). So it was good, and we plan to continue on with this over the next day or so. But the problem with automatic recording, so cheap and easy, is that you also risk talking much more—not merely than you can use, but than anyone's ever going to spend the time to review, let alone edit.

Paul arrived for a three-day jaunt. We spent the afternoon characteristically mixing dishing and working. Setting forth a definite short-term and general long-term publication strategy and a division of labor for that, how he'll edit the journals (John and Paul will tape-record me tomorrow and all this will be used as biographical background for the text).

But again, I mean, after all, who is she? Who, indeed, does she think she is? What possibly could justify all this attention? Paul said that once again he rushed to my deathbed to find me chipper, lucid, and even looking comparatively well. That seems to ignore that all through the day I was strapped to the bed being transfused, chemotherapized, and running alternate fevers and chills. There really is no material improvement, I still doubt this represents a reprieve. I told Paul I'd title this chapter of the journal, "As I Lay Dying . . . Again."

Sue Cramer was here and I read her the now almost completed paper that I didn't get finished for the IMA forum last week but she wants to publish. Given IMA's very limited circulation, I'd rather switch it with the Melbourne paper that Ross has for his Bicentenary volume [*Outer Site*], a paper which I hate and whose rampant sloppiness I don't know if I can repair. Shockingly, nobody seems to notice or care about that, and Robyn McKenzie wants it also for some new art tabloid. You get to wondering whether people actually read these things, or what they read, or why you spend so much time trying to get it right.

The oddness I keep describing for the experience of being so objectified (recorded, reviewed, evaluated, published) seems weirder and weirder. I'm sure I've gone way over the top of the allowable centimeter count for tall poppies (at least in my little Sydney world); they've got the axes oiled and ready, and even being so outrageously politically correct as dying of AIDS may not buy me another inch at this point. Paul has my stuff committed for the next 200 issues of *Art & Text*—says I'm cited ten times in the current issue, not counting Marcia's monograph review.

I'm only 40; most of the writing people cite doesn't go back more than five years. And I have no interest, as I'm sure and trust John and Paul don't, in invoking any lurid tabloid mythologies about "great potential nipped in the bud," or "AIDS: The tragedy of what he could have been. . . ." At least one reason for publishing this journal is to counter the sentimentalized narratives that seem to be all that San Francisco has been able to produce about this sequence; and to reconfirm first principles. But I can't help feeling uneasy and wonder if some etiquette or sense of style needs to be considered when agreeing to any, assumedly posthumous project, or the possible sum consequence of all this attention. (Though mustn't fool oneself about the size of the readership and range of circulation; we're definitely not talking household name here.)

When I mention this to John or Paul, for instance, they reply now with an analysis of how they see me as fitting, maybe even in some respects coincidentally, into what has (and hasn't) been going on in Australian intellectual life. And curiously, part of this is attributed to my coming from American traditions (similar to remarks O'Regan makes in his review [of *For a Cultural Future*]). So I've come full circle from my arrival when I was subjected to that impossibly contradictory challenge to prove I wasn't CIA (where the best proofs are identical to the best cover; and anyway, the real contradiction is everybody really hoped I was CIA, the left's romanticism having sunk that far). I reckon—and this has Warlpiri sources, too—that dying here does give me certain Australian "citizenship" rights. So there, Hon. Clyde Holding [new Minister for Immigration and former Minister for Aboriginal Affairs]!

June 22, 1988

I didn't even notice it was summer solstice until, unable to sleep last night, wound up from nonstop talk, I checked the 1 A.M. U.S. *Today* show on satellite feed and found Jane Pauley and Willard Scott making their little big thing about the first day of summer (followed by scenes of riots at Stonehenge!). One of I. B. Singer's stories is set in Argentina and comments on the difficulty that immigrant Jews had maintaining Pesach in the fall, Succoth in the spring, and so forth. Apparently, they just pushed on and went ahead; the Talmud doesn't seem to anticipate the antipodes. I myself could never sort it out, and this I hold responsible for my own deritualization and perhaps the entire Australian nation's.

John and I taped through to about 1979, but the chronology got jumpy. Austin and its complexity of social sites, cultural stratifications and sexual occasions during this period when it doubled in population, was not easy to describe. Nor was the anthropology department there. And anyway, there was a year spent in Philly and New York in the middle, and I didn't even mention John Weimer (or any of my other domestic dramas, for that matter). We got up as far as my thesis, but I'll have to do that with Paul, as John's off back to Sydney. I'm disappointed we didn't get to do the tape I thought was important—attempting to connect what I thought I was doing here and what my recent reviewers judge I've done. How we get from a 1960s American education in social science and philosophy to a "lionized" figure in Sydney critical debates deserves a go. And I don't think that one can be done as a monologue.

Penny and John passed each other at the airport. She and Paul went to dinner with Stuart C. (about which I feel some resentment as I feel Stuart's been neglecting me, just because he has a thousand papers to mark)—everybody seemed to get along fine, fortunately.

June 23, 1988

When my mother died, we received letters which recounted a specific anecdote or two of an episode the writer had shared with Mom. These were very touching, and I realized they represented a genre, but one I'd been completely unaware of (most examples came from our mostly Anglo friends; I don't think it's a Yiddisher thing). Well, now I'm getting similar letters, quite different from the lovely but more general support letters of several months ago that people sent when they first found out I was ill. I'm starting to have this odd sense of being at my own funeral. In fact, I've received simultaneously a shitload of the most spectacular (and expensive) flower arrangements wired in from all over the place so that I lie in bed feeling like I'm peering out of my own coffin. The current arrays all come from anthropology colleagues, and notably the most elaborate from people I've been having somewhat formal spats with. I wish gift horses wouldn't always insist on opening their mouths so bloody wide.

June 24, 1988

I have quite purposely resisted continuing to describe my analysis of the institution(s) of the Royal Brisbane Hospital and the outrageous contradictions of its discourses which I handled so brilliantly earlier in these diaries. I fear it too easily can be interpreted as whinging, inasmuch as it is redundant; that is, the contradictions just go on and on, not much new, but no less virulent. Having become productive again, I'm again impressed with how the place isn't just not set up for that, but resists it, tries to enforce passivity (unto death, I dare say!) so that to get any work done I have to work around and against the realization that I'm in a place that wants to kill me (even as my doctors—some of them—try to save me). But the staff seems impressed with my laptop, the very idea I'm working, the very classy look of my visitors, at least as much as the spectacular flower arrangements and the overseas calls. If I could only stop screaming at them every time they fuck up my medication (on average, twice a day) or try baby talk on me (only the new ones, but staff turnover is constant), we might get along okay. But I'm certain I'm at the top of the difficult patient list, exceeding even Chow the Chicken Man and the deaf and blind guy who can only communicate by moaning constantly as loud as he can.

More interesting, we finally got my will straightened out, I think. I'd gotten worried about it, and that I hadn't had a chance to go through it with John. But the copyright clause seemed ambiguous and it was completely unclear to me who owned what and who was empowered to make decisions about future publications. Paul was even more worried; my intent to give certain powers to Yuendumu might, for example, give them the right to block publication of these diaries, which seemed completely inappropriate, and the experience of the last issue of *Art & Text* and the graffiti business certainly was not reassuring. What if, in the most (not least) likely case, an arrangement is made to publish a collection of my [Aboriginal] art articles; am I really willing to let that be sunk because Neville or Chris have been born again, again, and don't like the illustrations, decide I'm a poof, a Jew, told I'm a commie, or even decide to repudiate their own traditional culture and happen to occupy a pivotal position in the WMA that year (assuming there is a WMA that year)? I really don't have much trouble admitting that my commitment to the principles of community self-determination is less than my determination to resist attacks from the Christian fundamentalist right.

Before, I was able to broker these issues face to face as I was accorded a persona and speaking rights over my five years of work and association with Yuendumu. But nobody else could do that for me or even be expected to try. And what if the old people—this is an unlikely scenario—decided to extend mortuary restrictions to me and my name: Am I willing to have everything withdrawn from circulation? "Well," I said to Paul and Penny, "I'm sure that if any of these things were to happen, it would spark such a productive debate in so many quarters that it would almost be as though my work were continuing even in my absence, and perhaps this would be more valuable than a few books could ever be, given how central I think these issues are to the chances for a cultural future." Talk's cheap. Do I really so unproblematically believe that any more? And at the very least, I think it's unfair, if not impossible, to expect anybody to serve as editor or publisher under such conditions of uncertainty, and that some compromise decision had to be reached. Also, though I retreated behind O'Regan's review of my work ("questions rather than answers") in defending myself to Penny and Paul, I had to admit that I needed answers here. Anyway, I asked Penny to go over the will with the lawyer and get this and a number of other bothersome questions clarified, such as: Where do profits go, should there be any from book sales? I thought they went to WMA. But did I intend for such things as the diaries (which by this time Paul is convinced will outsell Jackie Collins) to profit them?

It turns out that, yes, WMA could censor everything, but in fact got nothing for it all. By some incredible misunderstanding, Stuart and Lee got everything. Penny didn't even get expenses, and WMA only got to bellyache. I had Penny instruct Neil to void the will immediately, and replace it with one that gave everything to my estate, administered by Penny, instructed to take advice from John and Paul, household goods to Lee and Stuart, and was only able to get in a clause of advisement and consideration for WMA and the Warlpiri people of Yuendumu, which Neil even took it upon himself to reduce from my original wording (to continue a process of vetting and consultation negotiated in my lifetime). I'm a bit disappointed, wish I could do better, but am amazed at how much agro and time this involved given that there's almost no material property and no heirs/descendants involved. Maybe it's those unusual facts which are indeed the problem for the standard procedure. I sure hope Penny, Paul, or John don't get into any major disagreements. . . . I hope, I hope.

June 26, 1988

Sleepy today, quite exhausted. In fact, Lee came by. Nothing very interesting in the mail. Longish chat to Dr. K. I was pretty much right; I'm not going to some Rose Bay, $800-per-day private hospital around the corner from Paul overlooking the harbor, or anywhere for that matter. All my medications substitute for systems not functioning. They don't make them function. Should those systems (blood, lymph, immune) decide to start up of their own accord, well and dandy! And we'd be more than delighted (e.g., flabbergasted, though it's not beyond the realm of all possibility—something like that happened in November, but there was more of me left to work with then). That's today's medical update, diary dear. Nothing we could call an improvement except what is referred to by that nasty term, "quality of life."

Penny left after lunch yesterday. It had gotten a bit rough. My fevers were continuing, I was really drained from the work of the previous few days, and Penny had taken it upon herself to "sit up" with me. This is a curious ritual I'd forgotten, but in fact had not so long ago inflicted on my own poor dying mother. It assumes that the patient shouldn't be left by herself, and so somebody sits by the bedside, even beyond the point of having nothing to do or say. Of course, if the patient isn't in a coma, I suppose they can just ask to be left to sleep or something, but as ever, my misplaced sense of politeness intrudes and I'm afraid to offend. So again, I get irritable and subtly bitchy, and then maybe less subtly. Penny complements my problem here by supposing (I imagine) that because I'm so ill she can't tell me to fuck off, and she won't leave and abandon her responsibility. And so it goes: a classic, grotty Laingian "knot."

What's weird, thinking about it, is that I mostly get into these with women. Am I really a misogynist, then? In fact, it describes more generally the end point of every single live-in heterosexual couple I was in during my pre-gay youth, and I had identified the symptoms explicitly by my early twenties. I also noticed it didn't happen with guys, or at least in anything like the same way (the guys I was chasing in those days never turned around to chase me back, which I now think has a lot to do with all this). And most shockingly, at least some women seemed to sort of expect, even put up with, this sort of attitude/treatment from me. I assumed that once it had come to that constant sense of irritability (which my experience convinced me was irreversible), the game was over, *finis*, hit-the-road-Jack. . . . Nothing else good was going to happen. But I see something very similar depicted in recent documentaries about courtship, marriage, wife abuse, family law courts, and so on. Apparently, men and women irritate each other a lot (if my own folks did, they'd managed it, and it was invisible by the time I was old enough to possibly notice).

I thought the real source of this, my idiosyncratic problem, was that I was suppressing my homosexual desires—perhaps blaming it on women. When I was "reeducated," NYC, ca. 1972 (on the tail of another heterosexual affair gone irritable), by some curious logic I imagined I was actually taking the only possible course to overcome the blockage, and expected I would eventually be able to undertake a straight pair bond this way. Ha, ha! The truly grand irony, of course, took about six more years to hit me in the face like a wet bladder: the same thing could and did happen with guys (even butch ones).

This tangent may be prompted by my just getting off the phone with John; I already miss his company, and the above really is filling in some interstices in the tapes we were making.

In fact, Pen and I did manage to have some good fun with the camera. We took some night-flash "specimen" shots for Juan to work from for the portrait, but also some shots that might serve as graphics if needed. Saturday morning we went outside to the little garden and got more aggressive and elaborate. All nude to the waist down, featuring the cancer lesions most prominently. One shot in wheelchair, flowers in arms and hair. There goes Michaels, terrorizing the ward again!

My reservations about the etiquette of stage-managing my own posthumosity have obviously all been sunk. In for a pence . . . Paul always incites me to such scandal. And now I see the advantages of being merely a cult figure, writing for a specialized audience, circulating in these very restricted orbits. When I first started worrying about publicity of my illness, and the possible dreadful uses to which varying parties might put such news, by media I assumed the mass press. And in combination with the vulnerability of my immigration status, this has constrained certain of my choices, actions, even writings. In the most obvious example: Don't go to demonstrations where you might get arrested. But also, don't challenge that parking ticket, argue with the cop, lodge a noise complaint, write a letter to the editor, attract undue attention. Back in the closet again. . . . As frustrating as I sometimes found this (a situation all Queensland PWAS face, but to a shocking extent, healthy ones too), I have to admit there was some value in it; at times I could easily have gotten out of hand.

At the same time, of course, I'd been shooting for the highest visibility within my profession and on an intellectual circuit, and my survival seemed equally dependent upon doing just that; being seen to be continuingly productive, valued, important, even a star in what admittedly is a small firmament. And I pulled out a lot of stops that I never would have, at least at this point, if only because I don't think I would have really been interested in sustaining the effort to stay where a successful campaign of this sort is supposed to get you, while backsliding is a terrible (and too familiar) spectacle here at the Blue Angel.

That's what's so nice about non-mass media, and partly why some of us remain attached to its very limitations. It allows you this specialized, even subversive, circulation. So what if only 15 people heard my "Gay Waves" radio interview, or *Art & Text* is read by not many more (though we're lucky it's bought by more than that). These may be just the folks I wanted to talk to, and you can at least pretend that maybe they're a bit less likely to be the ones to turn you in to the mind police. But of course, there is an interface between the small-scale public media and the mass, and I'm never certain how or when this is activated. An interesting research project. But I think now I've escaped the worst of the possible consequences of being discovered (so longed for in my youthful quest for stardom) so that even if Paul is right that these diaries get a wider than cult reading, no worries mate! And that's why Juan can paint the cover and I can call the thing *Unbecoming* (though I still like *Should Have Been A Dyke*), and we can throw the whole bucket of blood up. I have the satisfaction, my anger transubstantiated.

June 28, 1988

Egad! My condition actually has improved. Most of my blood indicators are up substantially. This could actually require the scripting of an additional scene, or even act. I'm not all that pleased. In fact I've been lethargic and barely gotten out of bed, though I suspect I'm up to getting around quite well (the real test of my mood is whether I use the urine bottle or get up to go to the loo). I still have intermittent chills/fevers, but they seem to be coming under control.

Dr. K. discussed with me getting a desk or a file or something into the room so I can work and keep my papers in some kind of order. Obviously, I can't go back to the flat without a nurse. And I feel just too locked into this chemical factory to try and shift supports to Sydney no matter what.

Part of my mood is certainly anxiety over brother Mark's imminent arrival. Will we spat like six-year-olds? Will he Bible-bash me? And how shall I entertain him (everybody from Griffith's still fluey, and may be no help). One has certain obligations as hostess no matter what. Why is it that my definition of family is reduced to "people who can get away with checking for dust on the top of the bookshelf"?

June 30, 1988

Well, Mark turned out to be quite pleasant. Other than the unavoidable snaps of the family, there was none of what I feared, and we had quite a good chat for several hours, prompted by me, and mostly family gossip/reminiscence. In fact, I might try taping a recall session with him, though I'm becoming convinced that I've now exceeded what anybody's interest in my life could possibly be, and this excessive archiving should soon cease.

We went back to the flat so I could get Mark oriented. It looked very odd, perhaps anyway (as I'd never expected to see it again), but also as a result of tiny but perplexing alterations my recent guests have performed. How on earth can I still feel proprietorial about anything. But who left the cover off the mustard jar?

Today (and maybe tomorrow also) I have to go to school to direct the cleaning out of my office. They weren't going to bother me, I gather, just pack it all up in random order so that everything became subsequently irretrievable; which, admittedly, would have been the case if I was dead by now as we all expected, and conversely wouldn't have been a problem if I were more organized and less a slob generally. Still, I'd have appreciated more notice and I'm not really excited about having to undertake this right now. I'm glad Mark's willing to drive, and I'll appreciate his chauffeur services especially.

July 2, 1988

Cleaning out the office was less difficult but actually more taxing than I'd imagined. Haven't gotten to the files yet, but they look fairly in order as well. But I have to stop leaping out of bed with each new recovery as though I were instantly well and fully energetic again. Following two afternoons at school, I was completely buggered, couldn't get out of bed today, cancelled dinner with Stuart (Mark went solo), and generally felt shitty.

Mark has been thoughtful and helpful. But so far we've backed off from any very intimate discussion, even of the sort we began that first afternoon. I'm actually quite frightened of intimacy with him, and I can only make some guesses as to why. There is, as ever, my discomfort with my brother as flawed reflection of myself, and especially my judgment that he's stylistically "uncool" in precisely the ways I devoted myself to being "cool," and perhaps have failed to be, I suddenly fear, when I'm with Mark. There may also be a more particular history of suppressed episodes, a legacy of guilts, and so forth. In that first afternoon's chat, summarizing Jill's reading of our family, I told Mark, "Jill was Dad's, I was Mom's, and you always got the short end of the stick. Jill reckons as a result, she was brutalized and I was spoiled. You had the arguable advantage of being ignored." How much more deeply do I want to delve into any of this? It's oddly painful. And yet, it's quite clear that Mark is taking my situation quite hard in some way and it would be worse than unfair to ignore that or deny him some intimacy and some opportunity to talk about it.

July 3, 1988

I've been working my way through the AIDS issue of *October* that Paul sent. I was thrilled to receive it; I fancied this would put me in touch with all of the politics, debates, and analysis I've missed out on. About halfway through, I was less sure. I began to feel I was trudging through a swamp of discursivity, sinking deeper and deeper into a too-predictable rhetorical mud. Admittedly, the volume picks up midway when it shifts away from analytic deconstruction to statements by activists and PWAS, which I found moving, informative, and identifiable. In fact, the appeal from prisoners in the AIDS section at Rikers Island complaining about the pigeon shit on their windows blowing into the room wrecked me completely; these are the specificities that wipe us out in the end, and may prove harder to resist than any linguistic bias or the entire mass media apparatus.

Crimp's introduction is okay in that it raises the relevant question, "Can art fight disease, save lives?" But there is a subtle shift then to criticism, away from art; and in most of the academic pieces that follow, the appropriate question would have been, "Can deconstruction (e.g., Foucault and Derrida derivations) save lives, fight disease?" The articles themselves progressively veer away from that question. Instead, they mount a more general, if familiar, social criticism (mostly) of patriarchy into which the discourses of AIDS are demonstrated to fit quite nicely. This produces some handy statements about society, but I think its AIDS activism is pretty thin. We already know nobody likes faggots, and hardly expect late capitalism to show much sympathy. Worse yet, despite a sustained attack on victimization and the discourses of the afflicted, I wonder if a sort of liberal humanism infects these analyses, which, by exempting gays from criticism, in its own way renders us passive, and so victims in terms of our own arguments in the end. I stuck my tongue (and my arm, and my cock) into some pretty odd places during the 1970s, and remain unsure about some of that. Desire rarely proved to be democratic. We continued to police the class structure as much by our sexual choices as our careerism. Is there no way to discuss these things, to evaluate them and possible complicities in our present conditions outside the tacky theologies of guilt and retribution, or the sensationalism of Randy Shilts or the *National Enquirer*? Bersani's article ["Is the Rectum a Grave?"] is the welcome exception. But I think Paul is right (and should be encouraged) in his application of Sade to these questions, that Juan's hideous iconographies are important, and, in another way, that this diary and its publication are justified. I suspect that the academic half of this issue of *October* recapitulates for me my growing dissatisfaction, not merely with deconstruction and discourse analysis, but textuality as a subject/metaphor in general. Nothing especially original or new about these reservations (Foucault certainly expressed them). Even so, they may point to a certain sort of chutzpah in this issue that needs to be exposed.

July 7, 1988

Mark's gone, and I think the visit went well, for both of us. Having a chauffeur was a great help, obviously. But more, I'm surprised at how we were able to broach various difficult topics regarding, for instance, the family, Mom, Dad, and even our feelings and remembrances of each other. Mostly, this took place the last two days when I began to fear that I was keeping my distance in a manner not unlike what I criticized Dad for. But it was becoming more and more clear that Mark was profoundly moved, concerned, worried about my condition and imminent death, more so than I'd anticipated (or even thought about). His big brother owes him some reciprocal concern, I think. Classical melodrama requires some grand scene at this point in the narrative: a confession, a revelation, an accounting of some dramatic sort, which then makes comprehensible the whole plot out of which the family and its interior relationships are constructed. But we couldn't find a great deal to confess, and no such conventional ritual was enacted. Too bad, in one sense, because in cross-checking our recall of events, and filling each other in on recent ones, our family does look madder and more pathological than I'd been willing to concede. It would have been nice to have a pat melodramatic explanation to uncover. In fact, Mark had actually tracked down newspaper clippings about Grandpa Jesse's murder. . . . Intriguing, but not especially informative, apparently. It might suggest Mark is indeed seeking explanation for something, though more likely it's just a reasonable curiosity. I'd always wanted to know more about all that but was too lazy to do the research.

I'm pleased Mark and I accomplished what we did despite the persistent discomfort I feel with his style and presentation: the sense of being reflected in a flawed mirror. I was frequently irritable and withdrawn (partly due to my lack of energy and the expenditures required). Mark was tolerant. But he's so bloody American! So uncritical, unreflexive; we ate at McDonald's (my perverse choice, actually, but yes, he knew the menu by heart!). Oddly, this all reconfirms that part of my commitment to remaining in Australia—which is politically and intellectually based, as much as I'd like to go back if only to be relieved of constantly being an American, a foreigner, the Other, and subject to whatever anybody already thinks about that.

Martin sent me flowers from Melbourne. Stuart came by for a chat. The Toynes arrive tomorrow.

July 10, 1988

So weak. Everything's a chore (including writing in this diary). Richard reckons it may be due to taking me off the cortisone and expects my energy to return in 3–4 days now that he's restored the medication.

I drift in and out of sleep; there's really nothing else to do. As a result, I dream excessively, and the membrane between sleep and wakefulness is very porous, nearly translucent. Most dreams appear wholly trivial, as if I've used up the store of *significata* and only have random images now to assemble erratically. Waking up in the middle of the night, I return to a dream about Yoko Ono, mostly, methinks, because the line from the Lennon song "In the middle of the night I call your name" is incidentally invoked.

Sister Jill gave me *The Interpretation of Dreams* for a very early teenage birthday (14? 15?), a symptom I suspect of our sibling intellectual rivalry rather more than any endorsement of Freud. But as seminal a place as that text occupies in my intellectual history, I'm not sure that then or now I've quite accepted its major premise, and some central tenets of Freudianism. I have trouble identifying a Freudian theory of the social; it all seems essentially atomistic to me, which, to my way of thinking, problematizes any social models of communication.

Dreams employ all of the apparatus of communication, and we talk about dreams as communicative (and therefore social) acts even though it is unclear who, or what, is communicating to whom. From this angle, dreaming itself would seem to drive the last nail into the coffin of any dyadic model of message transmission, requiring a reconceptualization of all communication—not just dreams—as arising from social, not individual, territory. This would get us on a course closer to my own biased thinking (perverted, notably, by Ray L. Birdwhistell's 1973 Annenberg seminar) and away from at least some of the assumptions reified in our language and culture.

By partitioning the person into not merely diverse functions but contrasting selves, Freud offers an out which appears to get around this problem and can be employed to preserve the dyad (and the mystification of the individualized self). The id, for example, can be thought to be communicating with the ego, one acting then as sender, one receiver, and thus avoiding the problem of the social that I suggest dream communication poses conceptually. Although bulky, as solutions go, it seems to work to the extent that today most people believe something like it. One needn't know Freud to assume that a dream is a message sent from one part of oneself to another, and to seek its interpretation in that way. Alternately, one may think of dreams as messages sent from someone (somewhere?) else to the self: a god, an ancestor, a mere acquaintance. This is probably still believed by many (maybe most) people, but is considered too metaphysical for polite intellectual company. I agree, and submit that a fundamentally different sort of thinking is required. But the metaphysical explanation may yet be more helpful to achieving this; e.g., how does decentering the dreaming subject deconstruct—and radicalize—dyadic models?

This is a problem with journal notes. They're only halfway thought through, and liable to reveal as much ignorance as anything else. I certainly wouldn't venture a paper, even a lecture note on this subject. What do I mean by "seminal" after all, other than I haven't read *The Interpretation of Dreams* for 25 years? But here, I still wish to impress, to cloak myself in an appearance of insight—more, I admit, of range than depth, let alone precision. Or I'm just trying to extrude some retroactive value from a series of hopeless days in which my mind wandered and my motivation, not to mention my insight, were nil.

Incidentally, the status of my illness is rarely clear (let alone a topic) in my dreams. I have to review, on waking, to determine whether my

KS was visible to others, whether I was incapacitated in any way, whether I scared people, whether I flirted, or even attempted sex. Usually, but by no means always, I am not visibly ill. Curious! Curious also that I don't judge my condition directly, for example, by my capacity for physical exertion (do I run a mile? swim the harbor?), but by others' response to me and my appearance/behavior.

* * *

[*The following letter is discussed in the next entry. It was supplied by the executor of Eric's estate as an essential document missing in the diary.*]

Ms. Linda Anderson
South Brisbane Community Legal Service Inc.
PO Box 143 West End QLD 4101

Dear Ms. Anderson

RE: DR. ERIC PHILIP MICHAELS

I refer to Dr. Michaels' application for Resident Status on the basis that he fulfilled the conditions of sub-section 6A(1)(d) or 6A(1)(e) of the Migration Act 1958 and must inform you that it has been refused.

The decision has been made by an officer authorised under Section 6A of the Migration Act 1958 with reference to Government policy after careful consideration of the information you and Dr. Michaels have provided and the merits of his application. The reasons for refusal are outlined in the attached copy of the record of decision.

The authorised officer also considered the question of Dr. Michaels' further stay in Australia as a temporary resident or visitor. He has determined that should a formal application for further temporary stay be lodged, if there are no new circumstances, then the application should be refused. The reasons for this decision are also included in the attached record of decision.

If after consideration Dr. Michaels is convinced that the decision to refuse the application is wrong, he may seek an independent review of the decision by the Immigration Review Panel.

A pamphlet explaining how to exercise his right of review is enclosed. Should he decide to appeal, a copy of this letter should be attached to the request for review which must be lodged within 28 days of the date of this letter or the right of review will lapse. The application for review should clearly state the reasons or grounds on which he disputes the refusal of his application.

I should add that it is not proposed to seek the departure of Dr. Michaels from Australia while he remains medically unfit for travel.

Yours sincerely
Dario Castello
State Director
4 July 1988

DEPARTMENT OF IMMIGRATION,
LOCAL GOVERNMENT AND ETHNIC AFFAIRS
QUEENSLAND REGION

Minute

File No: 2405b
RES/JD:RLF

GRANT OF RESIDENT STATUS IN AUSTRALIA
ASSESSMENT REPORT

To: D. CROSSLAND
Director
Migration and Visitor Entry Branch

Purpose: To recommend that you:

(i) adopt the findings on material questions of fact and the assessment as set out below and refuse the grant of resident status to Dr. Eric Michaels (b) 11 February 1948 (40 years), a U.S. citizen, and

(ii) consider the question of granting a further temporary entry permit to Dr. Michaels. The question has been raised by Dr. Michaels and his solicitor although no formal application or fee has been received.

OUTLINE OF REASONS

Findings on Material Questions of Fact

1. PERSONAL PARTICULARS

Surname	Michaels
Previous Surname	n/a
Given Names	Eric Philip
Date of Birth	11 February 1948

Marital Status	Not Married
Citizenship	U.S. Citizen

2. IMMEDIATE FAMILY COMPOSITION/DISPOSITION

i) Australia	nil
ii) United States of America	Father, 2 siblings
iii) Elsewhere	nil

3. IMMIGRATION HISTORY

Dr. Michaels entered Australia as a Temporary Resident (code T23) on 31 October 1982. He was employed as a Research Assistant with the Australian Institute of Aboriginal Studies in Canberra.

On his arrival he was granted a 3 year 'unrestricted' temporary entry permit valid until 31 October 1985. Dr. Michaels was granted further temporary entry permits valid to 28 February 1987 to enable him to continue his work and consider a number of job offers.

4. APPLICATION FOR THE GRANT OF RESIDENT STATUS

Dr. Michaels lodged the application for Resident Status on 27 February 1987 and paid the prescribed fee (Q - fol 2). The application was made under Section 6A(1)(d) of the Migration Act relating to occupational grounds.

I have read all the material presented. There are no grounds for consideration under Section 6A(1)(a), Section 6A(1)(b) and Section 6A(1)(c). I find some claims relevant to consideration under Section 6A(1)(d) and Section 6A(1)(e).

The applicant's claims:

1) Dr. Michaels' claim for Resident Status on 'Occupational grounds' i.e. s6A(1)(d) was based on his 'continuing appointment' to a Senior Lecturer position in the Humanities Department at Griffith University. This appointment was subject to Dr. Michaels passing the University medical examination and him being granted Resident Status in Australia.

2) Subsequent claims put forward by Dr. Michaels, and on his behalf, regarding further stay in Australia have centred on his wish to remain here to continue his specialised work. Dr. Michaels has spent over 5 years in Australia working with Aborigines and researching the effects of introducing television to outback Aboriginal Communities. This work could not be carried out in the USA and is not applicable there.

3) Further, Dr. Michaels is suffering from Acquired Immune Deficiency Syndrome—AIDS—and it is not anticipated that he has more than 12 months to live. Dr. Michaels would like to continue his work in the time left to him. He has also stated that since his arrival in Australia his medical insurance in the USA has lapsed. He has claimed that if returned there he would not be in a financial position to pay for his medical treatment.

5. EVIDENCE OR OTHER MATERIAL ON WHICH FINDINGS ARE BASED

In reaching the above findings I had before me the following material:

- Department of Immigration, Local Government and Ethnic Affairs, Australian Capital Territory file number 82/19555 (folios 1–47), New South Wales Regional Office file N87/1049 (folios 1–5) and Queensland Regional Office file number Q87/18 (folios 1–122).
- Migration Act 1958
- Migration Regulations
- Grant of Resident Status handbook
- Migrant Entry handbook
- Department of Immigration and Ethnic Affairs
- "Health Standards for Permanent or Long-Term Entry or Stay in Australia—Guidelines for Australian Government Medical Officers"
- Legal and Policy Requirements for the Grant of Resident Status in Australia (M689)
- Department of Health report dated 6 May 1988 (fol 115).

6. ASSESSMENT

With the guidance of policy I have carefully considered the claims of the applicant, and I assess them as follows:

6.1. It is noted that Dr. Michaels was in possession of a valid temporary entry permit which permitted him to work at the time his application for the grant of resident status was lodged and consequently he met the legal pre-requisites of Sections 6A(1)(d) and 6A(1)(e).

6.2. In support of Dr. Michaels' original application on occupational grounds he submitted a copy of an offer of 'continuing appointment' to the position of Lecturer in the School of Humanities at Griffith University. The offer was subject to Dr. Michaels obtaining residence and successfully completing a medical review (fol 30/31).

6.3. Subsequent to the lodgement of the Resident Status application, Dr. Michaels was diagnosed as suffering from Acquired Immune Deficiency Syndrome—AIDS. His condition has been confirmed in writing by the Royal Brisbane Hospital where he is currently receiving treatment (Q - fol 104).

6.4. Dr. Michaels was requested to undergo a medical examination in relation to his grant of Resident Status application on 17 December 1987. A completed medical examination form has not been returned to the Department.

6.5. The fact that Dr. Michaels has been diagnosed as suffering from AIDS means that he fails to satisfy the health standards to be granted Resident Status. This Department's handbook "Health Standards for Permanent or Long-Term Entry or Stay in Australia—Guidelines for Australian Government Medical Officers" states in paragraph 6.3.1 'Evidence of AIDS or a related condition is cause for recommending rejection.'

6.6. This stand has been supported by the Commonwealth Department of Health. They have advised in their report of 6 May 1988 that in addition to the very expensive health care costs Dr. Michaels will incur as his disease progresses, there is also the risk that Dr. Michaels could pass on the disease to others (fol 115).

6.7. I have considered the letter from the Royal Brisbane Hospital that Dr. Michaels' therapy costs for the next 12 months or so will all be borne by the State (Q - fol 104). I have also considered that, while it is true that Dr. Michaels has previously contributed to the cost of his medical treatment, the fact that when the State undertakes to meet all his medical expenses means that these costs will be borne by the general community. I have also considered that the treatment being offered to Dr. Michaels may eventually be at the expense of an Australian citizen or resident who may also be suffering from the disease or another patient who requires the intensive care equipment which Dr. Michaels will need at the later stages of his illness. I have also considered that Dr. Michaels has let his overseas medical insurance lapse which could cause financial difficulty for him obtaining treatment. I have considered, however, that Dr. Michaels' treatment is available in his home country; that there are organisations set up to coordinate and provide assistance to AIDS sufferers, such as the National AIDS Network in Washington; and that all of Dr. Michaels' family are resident there.

6.8. In the applicant's favour I have considered that during the 5 years that Dr. Michaels has been resident in Australia he has completed numerous research papers on his work with Aborigines. The benefits of his studies to Australia and the Aboriginal Community has been attested to by the Australian Institute of Aboriginal Studies, Griffith University and the Australian National University and I believe we should fully accept the value of his contributions and give them considerable weight. I have also considered that during his time in Australia Dr. Michaels has contributed financially to Australia through the taxes he has paid, including the Medicare levy. Consequently it can be argued that Dr. Michaels has a right of access to the Public Health system.

6.9. On balance though I do not see that the factors weighing in favour of approval outweigh the possible health risks for the general community and the considerable public health costs which will accrue from the treatment given to Dr. Michaels.

6.10. Further I have considered that the Department has an obligation to protect Australian health standards (para 6.1.1 of Grant of Residence handbook refers) and that to allow Dr. Michaels to stay in Australia would be contrary to that obligation.

6.11. Dr. Michaels has also raised the question of further temporary stay in Australia though no formal application has been lodged.

6.12. Factors weighing in favour of approval have been stated previously and I accept they are relevant to a continued temporary stay.

6.13. Again, weighing against approval for further stay is his inability to meet the required health standards, the very expensive health costs which will be borne by the whole community in treating him, the use of health equipment and medical resources—possibly at the expense of an Australian citizen or resident—and the health risks involved with this dangerous disease.

6.14. I do not see that Dr. Michaels' personal circumstances are strong enough to warrant setting the health requirement aside and granting him a further temporary entry permit.

7. RECOMMENDATION

It is recommended that:

(i) the application for the grant of resident status to Dr. Michaels be refused, and

(ii) should an application for a further temporary entry permit be lodged, if there is no change in circumstances, then that application should also be refused.

J. Donnelly
Position No 6023
Resident Status Section
2 June 1988

Grant of Permanent Resident Status ~~approved~~ / not approved
Recommendation regarding the grant of a further temporary entry permit ~~accepted~~ / not accepted

D. Crossland
Director
Migration and Visitor
Entry Branch
Brisbane
3 June 1988

July 12, 1988

Letter from Immigration (via my lawyer) rejecting my visa application and, by implication, sending me home—wherever that might be. A dreadful and insulting document. Its illogic seems, at least to me and the lawyer, so obvious, its facts so flawed, that this would be evident to anyone reading it. A procedural response, capable of stalling any action, will probably cover the problem for a few months; a remark that I would not be deported while too ill to travel probably means never (though it puts a hard lid on my fantasies of going to Sydney).

July 13, 1988

Wretched. Sleepless night. Tried remembering every house or apartment I'd ever had (surprised how often I was living with other people or in other people's places). And got into some obsessive reminiscence about the Cullers, their house in Philly, and my last visit to them in

Marin. I suppose I fancy they should have been my parents (then I would have been Jonathan, I suppose). Not sure why I'm so determined to stay off Valium. If this happens again, I'll surely request one.

Stuart came over in the afternoon and took me out to Newstead House, but I was too weak to walk or do anything. Nick Z. came around in the evening; what a faithful visitor he has turned out to be. We rambled on about various topics, as we often do, for about two hours. In fact, we discussed this diary at length, and the limits of its reflexivity, Peter Ackroyd's fake Oscar Wilde autobiography. . . . What is a faux bon mot anyway? Jameson's piece on video, Nick's reply (but then Jameson is Jameson and Nick isn't, a fact whose postmodern significance, until Nick fully appreciates it, will disqualify his critiques and obscure the humor he intends so that it reads as mere pedantry). After about two hours, walking Nick out to wait for a cab, I had the most unpleasant and frightening experience: I couldn't get the intended words out of my head and through my mouth. It was utterly impossible to say, "John Lennon and Yoko Ono." Either nothing came out, or rubbish did. I could detour to a limited extent, and get out a sentence or two about something else. But the effect recurred and I'd be stuck on something else. I retired to bed with a nasty headache, hoping the effect was a product of overexertion and low blood pressure.

Reporting this to the new registrar (who I find easiest to keep at a distance), he pronounced that I had described exactly the symptoms of a form of aphasia which might be expected to occur resulting from lesions affecting the brain. Oh goody! Blood tests tomorrow and a CAT scan next week when a booking is available on the machine.

July 16, 1988

Still weak. Have been reading, reading, reading . . . books people drop off for me. What? Why? Who is Margaret Drabble? What do I care. Current British fiction all seems to be about real estate speculation to me, anyway.

July 18, 1988

Not much stronger, but I was going crazy and took 24 hours at home, looking forward to sleeping in Sunday morning. Stuart came by and took me to a faculty going-away barbie for Martin T. at Nick's new (quite charming) cottage. I think it's good form to show up at such things as long as I'm drawing salary. Even though I just sat and people came to me for chat, I found it quite draining and feared I'd not make it back up the garden steps at all gracefully when it came time to leave (except I did). Got home hopelessly weak. Spent Sunday morning on the phone to everybody before taxiing back to hospital.

July 19, 1988

Sue Cramer visited and gave me, among other presents, the current copy of *Artlink* with all the Aboriginal/Warlpiri stuff. I'd been warned that I'd hate Marcia's piece (opening address from Adelaide Arts Festival) so maybe that's why I didn't. She's absolutely stuffed when it comes to theorizing representation, but she does appreciate the on-site politics which are involved in art making/marketing, which may be at least as important in accounting for the work. What drove me wild was Megaw et al.'s piece, in which (perhaps through no fault of their own—one suspects they've been fed this news) they accord Françoise Dussart the credit for beginning acrylic painting on boards with the women at Yuendumu, which the men then copied.

It will be difficult to respond to and correct these factual errors without being seen as territorial, childish, or competitive—postures which Françoise draws me into all the bloody time! But there are facts, as well as motives at stake here; it scares me to watch the creation of false histories. The matter may not be as trivial as it seems at first. A kind of appropriation is involved whenever anthropologists insert themselves as mediator/interpreters and now helper/originators. In this way we don't merely discover, we do actually invent our tribes.

For the record: As I (and I think others) recall it, Françoise did indeed supply boards and paints to the women to reproduce the body painting designs she was then studying for her thesis on women's dance. In so doing, she was not doing much more than Nancy Munn had done collecting for her *Warlbiri Iconography* here 20 years ago, or the Berndts did in Arnhem Land, or many other ethnographers. In any case, acrylic paintings on boards had been done at Yuendumu for years, and could occasionally be bought at the Mining Company. Frank Baarda tells the story; apparently, they were regarded as crude and never sold very well to the occasional passing tourist. I'm not sure whether Françoise's women's studio preceded the men's work on the doors [of the Yuendumu school] or not; I remember them as being about the same period, but this hardly matters really.

Any claims to innovation in the Yuendumu case would have to account for: (1) the marketing/distribution strategy which was developed by the foundation of the Warlukurlangu Artists Association, which assured that painting could become a worthwhile and rewarding enterprise on an on-going basis (in terms of supply of materials, receipts, as well as prestige); and (2) the acknowledgment of something worthwhile (and marketable) in the "Yuendumu Style"—bright, "nontraditional" colors, an asymmetrical, Neo-Expressionist ("untidy") technique. In both these respects, Mlle. Dussart can take no credit. She fought us tooth-and-nail on both fronts.

That's why I do like much of Marcia's article. It highlights what I also think is so important: the creation of community-controlled art cooperatives and credit accorded to anybody who assisted in that always difficult undertaking, whether they ever supplied a canvas, brush, or not. Any "origins" must be dated from that. By contrast, Françoise sold the paintings on a personal, ad hoc basis, mostly to A.N.U. friends during her trips down south. So the distribution was entirely dependent upon her. Okay: but when Warlukurlangu got going, she refused for some time to give up on her "private" sales and caused quite a problem for documentation and simply keeping track of receipts, what was going where, etc. Likewise, she continued to insist on a dogmatically restricted "traditional" palette, and we had frequent arguments over whether the women should be allowed blue and green pigments. What emerged (and was marketed) as "Yuendumu Style" hardly can be credited with these origins! The worst part may be that Françoise (and Chris and Peter) have no concept of any of this, would find this argument quite alien, fail to recognize not only the dreadful politics of their claims, which demean the artists, but also reject the critical role played by Peter Toyne, Mark Abbot, and everybody else who worked their asses off to get a community arts organization going capable of sustaining a painting workshop. Françoise never could see the community in light of its contemporary situation; she seemed always to see things through the blinders of her peculiar ethnographic present. Now that this fantasy is being transferred wholesale to the South Australian Museum and inscribed in *Artlink* (as well as lord knows how many show catalogues), I think some response must be attempted.

July 21, 1988

Reading Anaïs Nin's last diary (1966–74) turned out to be a fairly unpleasant chore. It's so long ago since I read the earlier ones that I can't recall if they were much better. It is not simply her egotism in this last volume that is insufferable. But then, no dummy, Anaïs is quite articulate about this very point. She contrasts the aims of Eastern philosophy (denial and the submersion of the ego) with the goals of psychotherapy (the acknowledgment, articulation, even celebration of the ego) and recognizes that as a psychotherapist, she is somewhat out of synch with the times and even her own fans. Interesting point; certainly, I am more a child of Zen than of Freud. Of course, Nin could get away with her extreme self-assurance. As I remember her at her lectures at Temple University in 1972–73, she was so striking: 70-years-old, totally poised, even sexy, tiny and frail, but full of power. My complaint concerns what her egotism identifies as worth recording in the diary, what she sees as important, or at least telling enough to include; not to mention a certain racism that colors her accounts of her trips to exotic climes. And also, her idea that because her diaries are credited by some readers with having prevented them from suicide, their ultimate worth is established.

But, the reading still provided an eerie chronology to superimpose on my own reveries. 1966–77 were, for me, the critical moment of course, and I have been spending a lot of time reconstructing my past as I lie here, listless and otherwise bored. I'd hoped that certain correspondences between my circumstances and Nin's would also be interesting. The diary begins with her finally achieving recognition/fame, as I, in my much more modest way, now experience the beginnings of a limited celebrity, and the diary ends on her meditations on her cancer and impending death. Yet, instead of finding many useful insights or parallels, I find myself again consumed with this sort of confused envy which infects me all too often. Why did I grow up in so much more a Jewish bourgeois world? Why were my folks so stingy? Why have I been so peripheral to the scenes that attract me? Why don't my books get proper distribution? Why didn't I go to a more prestigious college? Why don't I have a Bleecker Street flat or Lloyd Wright house and swimming pool in the Los Angeles hills to expire in?

And then, Stuart shows up with a ton of mail from school, letters from Horace and Bob in Austin and Crocker in London and even unknown fans, and I am vindicated again.

July 24, 1988

Dallas is back on air, and I stay up Tuesday nights to watch. Pam is dying, dying, dead. It's so clever how they keep their characters going even into the next season after the actual actors have quit. In this case, Pam who blew herself up while talking on her car phone at the end of last season (only they don't really have seasons here in Oz—TV or climate—as they show the series in whatever slot and sequence their loony programmers dictate, unmoored from any rhythm of pseudo-immediacy, which makes all this seem like "current affairs" overseas) is now a huge, immobile white blob of sticky-tape lying in a hospital bed in Dallas Memorial, which is nowhere as posh as the hospitals in *Dynasty*. Her recovery is signified by her squeezing Bobby's hand. I presume "her"; we have no certain clues as to who or what may actually lie under all that tape, animating that response. Then suddenly she dies, as we knew she must, because Victoria Principal had quit the series some time ago, and they certainly weren't going to pull that trick they tried with Miss Ellie by substituting some other actress, which was a disaster. So, the only suspense left in much of the series now is methodological: just how (and when) will they bump off a character. Pam didn't really get much mileage here, but after her "it was all a bad dream" radical deconstruction a few seasons ago, she's entitled to a more modest retirement.

But *Dallas* doesn't really serve the functions that I seek in it any more. I don't get the sense of participating in a simultaneous, vast ritual of viewership linking me to the whole electronic world. Partly, this is because the programmers don't understand this function (and this attraction) of the blockbuster mega-serial. They are slack, even unconcerned about when they put *Dallas* to air here in Australia. Not only what night of the week, but what episode in sequence and time. Each state may be watching a different episode, be at a different point in the story, so that no sense of connectedness to anything larger than a regional audience is possible. How can you call Australia a country if everyone is at a different place in the story? States' rights gone mad. Consequently, TV here enforces, and does not collapse, distance. My wish to be in some quasi-mystical union with *Dallas* audiences everywhere—and in particular Horace and Jackie and Jim and others, who, though geographically dispersed, I know are watching the current episode wherever they are—is defeated.

July 25, 1988

John shot through between Sydney and Cape York where he's off to make a dance video with Dreadful Drid. He's not over his flu and I felt a bit worried for him. Good to see him, even if we had to keep it light. After all, it will be at least five weeks before he finishes at Edward River/Aurukun and we might spend some time together again. And frankly, I am less than enthusiastic about soldiering on much more, certainly not here in Wattlebrae Ward. John did get me out for the day and it was fairly taxing. We went over to Athol's in the morning and then napped back at my flat (I finally got my clothes out of the washer and up on the line!). Then off to McDonald's for late lunch—how perverse!—and then back to hospital.

July 27, 1988

". . . she fainted on cutting into a tomato for the first time in her life during the German Occupation." So far, Patrick White's best line in *Flaws in the Glass* and I'm already halfway through. How can he call himself a closet queen? In press? Penguin, no less? A contradiction in terms, which White is so full of, like his "republican" complaints in the sequel about having to go visit the royal yacht. But I read this stuff not only because Stuart leaves it for me, but because there is some insight here, about Australia perhaps more than homosexuality, although maybe mostly the strange intersection that occurs between the two.

Watched the SBS-TV doco *Living with AIDS* last night. Disappointing. Very Canberra-political: lots of hemophiliacs. Poofs at meetings, looking concerned, only one gay victim. It was good to see him, though, poised at the piano with the family snaps on the lid, playing "More" for all he was worth, smiling bittersweetly through his lesions. Like the first time I recall seeing KS matter-of-factly on TV, this was good, even if it slightly blows my cover (but only slightly; this is merely SBS). And after all this, Health Minister Blewett comes on to remind me that we (gays, IV drug users, hemophiliacs) are not members of the "general public"—a point which gnawed at the program's entire text but was hammered home dreadfully in Blewett's usage, despite his overt and explicit sympathetics. Is this intentional deceit? Or prejudice so deeply seated that he and the entire production crew don't realize the damage this causes? Maybe one can expect no more from liberalism. But it's exactly this that allows the Immigration Department to treat me so brutally and prejudicially. I wonder what really will or can happen if they try to move against me? I have no plans as yet, and am only now beginning to circulate their letter to my allies.

July 31, 1988

Transfusion. Richard started the drip at 8 A.M., thinking I could be through by noon. But it didn't finish till six. Dugald came over with raw cashews. We talked about the [Labor] government's white paper on higher education and the implications for Griffith—who we will teach, how, and even what. Nobody seems much concerned, oddly. Dugald says they're too involved debating the more local issue of a chair in media studies.

August 1, 1988

The transfusion mostly worked; I can get up and around, though my legs aren't quite used to it. I should get a week or two of functioning out of this. Spent yesterday on Stuart's verandah eating salt bagels with lox and cream cheese. Nick came by with a fabulous strawberry torte. After dinner watched a Schwarzenegger video with Jo and Ben. How deliciously normal a day in my Uncle Eric mode.

August 7, 1988

An official investigation has determined that the Iranian jetliner was blown up and 290 people killed due to "human error." Three people were killed and five injured yesterday when a hunk of a skyscraper under construction crashed into the main pedestrian mall here in Brisbane. Do not wonder that these diaries mostly ignore current events.

Michael Dukakis? Who cares. However, Pam turns out not to be dead after all. She had herself spirited out of hospital by the board chairman of Wentworth Oil to some hidden destination. She left a note explaining that when they took the bandages off she was so ugly she didn't ever want Bobby or little Christopher to see her. So she has abandoned husband, child, family, business that they may remember her instead as ever beautiful. Ignoring that the logic is so unbearably egotistical that we may never want to see Pam again anyway, the narrative move is merely another in the great *Dallas* tradition, which allows for maximum future hedge-betting. Pam now can come back in some undetermined future; she's only on hold for now. In fact, she can have plastic surgery and come back different. Somebody beside Victoria Principal can play her. Something like that was tried last season when this guy showed up claiming to be Jock. Nobody bought it—except Ray and Miss Ellie. The public sure didn't. So they put him in jail. *Quantum* had a BBC program on near-death experiences. They turn out to be the limbic system's response to oxygen depletion. But the experience of "seeing yourself" proved harder to explain. Could we always be seeing ourselves, in some Lacanian sense, but masking it, and perhaps other perspectives as well, so that finding yourself up on the ceiling is merely an unmasking? I certainly have spent a good deal of my life on the ceiling, I think.

You don't watch television in hospital; you surrender to it. I haven't quite yet, but that's partly, I'm sure, because the set I've inherited is so hard to watch and I'm too cheap or lazy to replace it (though actually, I depend on the alienating effect of poor reception).

August 8, 1988

Penny writes from Britain thanking me for being so uncomplaining. It seems her dying mother, by contrast, is being a terrible bitch and won't even let her out of the house to visit friends or anything on the basis of her having paid for the airfare. I'm not uncomplaining at all, though I try to be selective of whom I complain to. I'm quite put out by everything at this point, and don't really understand the virtue of attaching this tedious postscript to my life and work. In fact, I'm becoming resentful of this diary, Paul for making me write it, and the reader, assuming there is any willing to plough through all this, for requiring additional text. Why bother . . . ? Any of us? What's worth writing about? The trivia of my movements (bowel or otherwise) since the last entry? The indignities imposed on me by institutions? That now I'm going bald (and am still picking hair out of the computer keyboard)? The continuing horrors of the hospital? What I watched on TV today?

It's not that this can't go on. It seems it can, indefinitely. But like the bridges of New York City, the infrastructure begins to fall apart: traffic fines, unanswered letters, immigration—all the things I had only short-term solutions to, or thought I could ignore, are catching up again, and I just don't have any plan B's or the energy to construct them. Will they really drag me out of bed and off to jail? Or put me on an airplane to nowhere? I don't want to find out. Less and less of this drama interests me. I thought I'd done a reasonable job, announced my retirement a few months ago, but I'm still here, damn it!

August 10, 1988

Philip called from Alice. He is the proud father of Ruby Lucy something Tamara something. Everybody seems delighted. She's already been "smoked." Marcia and he seem to be managing together, a relief to be sure. Lots of good local and bushie gossip. Jim B. was there just back from the Hobart AIDS conference. He tells me about this Michael somebody from San Francisco who has been at terminal stage for three years and, with massive doses of Bactrim, treats it merely as a chronic illness, and keeps on keeping on. I told Jim I didn't know if that seemed such an attractive prospect, staring yet again at the blank walls of Wattlebrae as I spoke. Then, after the phone call, I thought: Why not go to Alice Springs? Even if I die getting there, the project still has more style than lying here and being bored to death. There really are a full dozen people there who would take on some responsibility for me, the AIDS group is Jim and my friends, the aesthetics are appealing—it would sure be cheaper than Sydney. So I indulged a fantasy of Bucknall driving me out, lying in the back of the station wagon, watching the desert go by again, getting to Alice Springs and receiving in state for the few weeks left. Even if by doing this I cut off a few possible days or weeks extra, it seems worth it. I sure can't motivate any optimism for continuing on like this here in Brisbane, but a few extra weeks might seem worth it in Alice.

The reason why not, of course, is the Immigration Department.

They've contacted Richard asking for a report of my condition and whether I'm ready to travel. Can you believe this? I was up all night drafting imaginary letters to everybody possible. Even a Valium couldn't help. They really insist on hounding me to death, and expect, perhaps correctly, that from my hospital bed I won't be able to muster the resources to do anything about it. They would be right only if I had any choice. But if I leave Australia, not only do I die, but I do so in some horrible, confused, totally alienated public welfare environment, with no friends, no confirmation of my life and work—just hysteria, rather than any possible satisfaction, fulfillment which anyone, any human, I think, is entitled to at death's door. Why would even the meanest bureaucrat be party to so mean a treatment? I still believe something can stop this madness, even if it takes getting Nugget Coombs to camp out on Holding's doorstep until the situation is resolved (though I could be mistaken; this has already gone further than I thought it possibly could). But even if it is resolved, the problem keeps me up at night, consumes what energy I have for writing and planning, hijacks all my agendas and otherwise completely overtakes these last days. That people willing to do this exist staggers me. That they can represent the official arms of the state depresses me more than I can say, or think.

* * *

[*Among Eric's papers was found the following untitled text. Nothing is known of its origin or purpose except that it seems to have been written in 1982, around the time he moved to Canberra from Austin, Texas. It is included here as an apostil to certain remarks made in the diary about defining gayness, gay political sensibility, and the prehistory of contemporary gay culture.*]

* * *

When we express our disappointment that gay life here has become apolitical, we conjure up an image in the minds of our younger friends of wild-eyed radical transvestites and hairy hippy faggots battling the forces of authority. It is not merely that we are seen as sentimental antiquarians, but worse, we are sentimental about a period which seems to the young so thoroughly unattractive. Some clarification is in order.

The misunderstanding seems to revolve around just what it means to be "political." For some of my generation, politics was indeed an activity: dramatic confrontations which were purposefully shocking and offensive to the public. The slogan, "You think faggots are revolting? You bet we are!" was one of my favorites. But it was not entirely clear even then whether flaunting our offenses at the middle classes was especially productive. It was fun, but that's another story.

More to the point, we developed what might be called a "political sensibility," and it was this that we valued so much. Sensibilities are difficult to define, but it seems important, here in 1982, to recall what faggotry was up to ten years ago, in thought as well as deed. First, we need to remember that a generation ago, say 1960, homosexuality was thoroughly illegal, unquestionably immoral, and was treated as such by society and its laws. Enlightened people advanced the liberal idea that we were *sick*, a big step up from criminal status. Instead of being arrested—and we were, often—we might be cured. In 1960, there were only two operating gay bars in New York City. I'm talking about only 22 years ago! It must be difficult for someone in their twenties now, who has been to this, or other gay meccas, to imagine such a thing. But this whole gay world, the discos, the bars, the magazines, baths and bookstores, are essentially a recent invention. Today, one can live almost completely in a gay society, spend our time, day in and day out, in gay-oriented shops, restaurants, laundromats, jobs, and never even notice that there is a society out there, let alone that it might disapprove. It isn't surprising that people growing up in such a world hardly feel the need to develop much in the way of a criticism of society. For that's what the gay political sensibility was; a critical perspective on American life and values.

These perspectives, and the criticisms, were quite varied; don't get the impression there was a party line. A visit to any gay meeting—rap group, consciousness-raising, political or social salon—would provide ample evidence of the diversity of perspectives and beliefs. In fact, the movement probably deteriorated in part because so many people had so many theories about what was wrong, and how to set it right. Some were Marxists, some Democrats, some romantics (if there were any Republicans in those days, we didn't know about them). What was agreed was that there was something wrong with a society which oppressed people the way we were oppressed. And of course, this meant we shared something with blacks, browns, women, and other people who were not getting treated right by the Anglo, male-dominated world.

There is a history to be written about what exactly happened between now and then. Basically, it would probably explain how some gay people started to make money, usually by capitalizing on other gay people, thereby creating an economic possibility that didn't exist before. These people now own the gay media, the gay bars, baths and bookstores (they used to be owned by the Mafia, when they existed at all). And they have successfully advanced a Dewar's Profile image of the gay capitalist that didn't exist before. They sold it to the gay public, along with Nautilus, EST, and Coors Beer, and a critical, political sensibility would be damaging to their gay interests. So they discourage it. The young'uns at the nouveau preppie discos are taught to believe they are mainstream American consumers, no different from any other upwards socially mobile business major.

Well, what's wrong with that?

First of all, it isn't true. If and when we venture out of our lavender prisons, we may notice a world out there where a sizeable proportion of the population thinks we are a "problem," who would like to see us all disappear, and some of whom would like to help in that. But that's not what bothers me so much.

What bothers me is that being a faggot isn't very interesting anymore. When I walk into a disco, or a bar, or a baths, I don't feel I'm entering any kind of new age. I don't feel I'm on the frontier. We're not avant-garde any more. We're not avant anything. We imitate everybody else now. They don't imitate us.

I liked being deviant. Particularly in a world gone half-mad, and a society that values profits over people, being deviant may be surprisingly joyous, life-affirming, celebratory. Just because gay people are now permitted, in certain places under certain circumstances, to share in the profits, to become consummate consumers, doesn't imply an improvement in our lot. Does anybody really have fun at the bars (without expensive drugs)?

Becoming normalized may not be all it's cracked up to be. To wit, we seem to have lost our strongest suits—the art of conversation, of style, of grace, even our sense of humor, caustic and brittle as it sometimes was. We're nothing special now; we're just "singles." And there is nothing to unite us, let alone to talk about, except consumables, apartments, cars, and finally men. So we drink more, and do more drugs I suspect, and we risk turning into those Valium-crazed suburban housewives that shopping malls and split-level homes provide backdrops for.

Maybe the lunatic right wing will mobilize and we will have to drag ourselves out of this languor to protect ourselves and respond. Or maybe the Baby Boomers will eventually reach their sixties and, upon looking back, develop a more powerful criticism than any advanced so far. Or gay epidemic cancers and diseases will mean we will have to learn the art of conversation again. But wouldn't it be lovely if we could reclaim our lost community, our arts and our skills, of our own initiative, in response to our collective boredom. For starters, we need to take some responsibility for our own history, for conveying it to our young. It is not nostalgia. If one is going to go to all the trouble to be gay, one ought to do a more interesting and useful job of it. Models exist in our very recent past. They should be recalled.

Eric Michaels was an ethnographer and a theorist of visual arts, media studies, and broadcasting. At the time of his death he was a lecturer in media studies at Griffith University in Brisbane. He is the author of *Bad Aboriginal Art: Tradition, Media, and Technological Horizons.*

Paul Foss is the editor and publisher of *Art & Text*, and recently edited Paul Taylor's posthumous *After Andy: SoHo in the Eighties.*

Michael Moon is Associate Professor of English at Duke University. He is the author of *Disseminating Whitman: Revision and Corporeality in "Leaves of Grass"* and is coeditor (with Cathy N. Davidson) of *Subjects and Citizens: Nation, Race, and Gender from* Oroonoko *to Anita Hill* (Duke University Press, 1995).

Simon Watney is the author of several books including *Policing Desire: Pornography, AIDS, and the Media* and *Practices of Freedom: Selected Writings of HIV/AIDS* (Duke University Press, 1994).

LIBRARY OF CONGRESS CATALOGING-IN-PUBLICATION DATA
Michaels, Eric.
Unbecoming / by Eric Michaels ; new preface by
Michael Moon ; introduction by Simon Watney.
p. cm. — (Series Q)
First published in Australia in 1990.
ISBN 0-8223-2005-3 (alk. paper). —
ISBN 0-8223-2014-2 (pbk. : alk. paper)
1. Michaels, Eric—Health. 2. AIDS (Disease)—
Patients—Australia—Biography. I. Series.
RC607.A26M53 1997
362.1'969792'0092—dc21
[B] 97-7920 CIP